# Scrofulous Affections

AND

THE ADVANTAGES OF THEIR TREATMENT ACCORDING TO THE PRINCIPLES AND EXPERIENCES OF

# HOMŒOPATHY.

DESCRIBED AND DEMONSTRATED BY NUMEROUS EXAMPLES OF SUCCESSFUL CURES.

BY

Dr. H. GOULLON,
OF WEIMAR.

TRANSLATED FROM THE GERMAN

BY

EMIL TIETZE, M.D.

---

"A misunderstanding only can place the essence of Homœopathy in small doses."
B. Hirschel.

---

BOERICKE & TAFEL.

NEW YORK:
NO. 145 GRAND STREET.

PHILADELPHIA:
NO. 635 ARCH STREET.

*SHERMAN & CO.. PRINTERS.*

"ALLOPATHS content themselves but too often with a removal of the peripheric phenomena, while the essence of the disease, the living centre, as it were, from which the most various phenomena issue, remains unmoved in all its force, or is transposed to a locality still more dangerous.

"The Homœopath, on the other hand, after a careful search for the peripheric morbid phenomena, endeavors to pierce the centre of the disease itself, and destroy it by a remedy homœopathically corresponding to it.

"J. BAMBERGER."

# PREFACE.

On superficial consideration it might appear superfluous to write upon a subject sufficiently dwelt upon by the most different authors in homœopathic literature; to speak at length of a disease, to recognize which, in many cases, is no difficult matter for laymen, even. For here the question is not as to the establishment of a diagnosis by means of laborious and minute microscopical experiments, or as to researches for repugnant animal or vegetable parasites; on the contrary, scrofulosis moves among the crowd of mortals unveiled, clumsily and openly, impressing a seal upon its victims easily to be recognized.

Though the fear of this momentous dyscrasia is not so strong and intense, as that of its near relative, tuberculosis; yet the verdict of the physician, "your child is scrofulous," does nevertheless, not unfrequently occasion great anxiety. And it will afford much consolation to parents to know that their child may be freed from its evil by gentle means.

This gentle liberation, however, can take place only by the application of the homœopathic method of healing, and just here the advantages and invaluable blessings of the new doctrine stand out prominently.

In view of the enormous spread of scrofulosis, it is of the greatest importance to state those advantages, as well as to uncover, without fear or favor, the shortcomings, not to say crimes, of the old antiscrofulous method of treatment, and to acquaint the attending physician with the new remedies in a comprehensible and practical manner. To write a monograph on scrofulosis in this sense, from the standpoint of humanity, so to say, as well as of science, is probably not without merit. It may be that Prof. Leo's notorious and ominous word of "the scrofulous plebs" will gradually die out, and be forgotten, if only the mild, rational method of curing gains ground over the erroneous one favoring both degenerations, and increase of the evil. Then, the uninvited and obtrusive guest will certainly have to shorten his visits, and the inmates of huts and palaces alike fare much better. The panic fear of parents, as well as of children, at mentioning the words "scrofula," and "anti-scrofulous treatment," may be removed, and changed into hopeful confidence.

Although there is no scarcity of reports of homœopathic cures of scrofula and its many species, these reports, nevertheless, are scattered, and mostly forgotten; they are, likewise, of unequal value, and not all equally commendable for imitation. For the purpose of obtaining homœopathic antiscrofulosa of real worth, we will, hence, let pass in critical review those reports of cures from the first date of their appearance to the present day, and recommend only what has proved itself of practical value.

There are self-evidently, as we have stated above, complications of scrofulosis with other constitutional anomalies which, however, cannot be regarded here; since the doctrine of genuine scrofulosis itself presents to us a complete literature of its own. Moreover, the principal momentum of the whole treatise will have to be placed in that portion of it pertaining to therapeutics. For, of what good to the reader are hypotheses, however ingenious; what help does it afford him, for instance, to be told that, according to Arlt, photophobia, blepharospasmus, watering of the eyes in scrofulous ophthalmia (pustular ophthalmia) are said to be but the results of reflex-action which the irritation of the sensitive branches of the n. trigeminus exerts upon the ciliary, lachrymal and facial nerves; would he not prefer to know, rather, that homœopathy possesses remedies by which it masters these reflex-phenomena together with their original source, and what they are? Thus the possibility of a quick and useful application of the material presented, must be the leading tendency. Besides, no great importance is to be placed upon the principle of classifying the various scrofula-forms, if only none of them are forgotten that can be easily recognized, and thus are well-fixed on account of their sufficiently characteristic phenomena.

It appears most convenient and practical, probably, to observe, as I shall attempt to do in the following pages, a physiologico-anatomical order. Before, however, the general consideration regarding the origin and essence of scrofulosis, may find a place here.

# CONTENTS.

ON

# SCROFULOUS AFFECTIONS.

---

## I.

## GENERAL PATHOLOGY OF SCROFULOSIS.

SCHLEIDEN, the celebrated botanist, used to open his lectures by frankly confessing to his attentive audience that he did not know what a plant was. Something similar happens to pathologists regarding scrofulosis; for while some form an idea thereof that takes in too little, others entertain one comprising too much. And though the knowledge of this disease dates far back in ancient times, there is yet, at the present day even, neither a Virchow nor an Oppolzer able to point out the last, so to say, biological cause of this dyscrasia. Or is the definition satisfactory, to say that scrofula results from disturbances of nutrition, taking place where poor and badly-aired dwellings, unhealthy, non-nitrogenous food,* an effeminating way of living and other conditions begetting disease, show their deleterious influence? Do we not find this evil in all its innumerable manifestations even where the conditions mentioned are absent?

Indeed, in derision, as it were, of all theories, we see that constitutions entirely opposite, are affected by scrofulosis. Fleshy, bloated, full-cheeked, phlegmatic individuals are free from it as little as is the sanguine temperament with its slim, vivacious, warm-blooded (arterial) character. Children living in miserable, overcrowded dwellings, who, all the year round,

---

* Though it is certain that aninal food, even, calls forth a predisposition to serofula (Bazin, Jousset).

have to support life by potatoes, and other vegetable diet, fall victims to this dyscrasia, as well as do the pets of fortune, and were they of royal blood, even.*

And sea-baths, an atmosphere loaded with the most precious perfumes; tender game, extracts of the most strengthening kind; mineral springs most carefully selected; amusements and entertainments the most exhilarating, are not always able to arrest the progressing decline. And less so if scrofulosis appears as a hereditary evil; or if unsuitable marriages are contracted among near relatives; for, from such unions, forbidden as they were, by the most ancient legislation for reasons, undoubtedly, more philosophical than religious, arise the dispositions to mental disease, tuberculosis and scrofulosis.

Bazin says: The scrofulous have "something in excess," "quelque chose d'excessif." They are either too tall or too small; too bright or too dull; too fleshy or too lean; too pink or too pale; have either too craving an appetite, or none at all; are either too amorous or too cold. Unjustly, probably, Jousset calls this characteristic picture: "Un tableau oû la fantasie a sa bonne part."

But, as I have just mentioned, not only marriages among near relatives favor the development of scrofula, but also the descent from a scrofulous father or mother; in short, hereditability; or there is, as we are wont to express it, an organic predisposition to the disease in question. Many families exhibit the taint through many generations, as Schoenlein has proven of the Bourbons in France, and the Salis family in Switzerland. In fact, not only scrofulosis as such is inherited, but also its special form, *e. g.*, a scrofulous affection of the organ of hearing, in a similar manner as mental disease, in general, and in a special form (*e. g.*, as melancholy ending in

---

* In England scrofula is singularly called "king's evil;" because since the time of Edward the Confessor, the gift of healing it has been attributed to the kings of England. In Holland it is called Klieren, Kropzweeren; in France, ecrouettes, skrophules. The Greek spoke of *χοιράδες*, from *χοῖρος*, the hog; on account of the similarity existing between scrofula and a disease peculiar to hogs. Finally, the Romans, on account of the roundness of the swelling, which is one of its most characteristic phenomena, used the term *struma*, and designated by this word the whole dyscrasia. So Celsus in his time. The term proper, scrofula, is derived from skropha (*γρομφάς*), the sow.

suicide), not rarely transplants itself hereditarily from one individual to another. With regard to the question, whether scrofulosis be communicated by the father or mother, Cullen says that the children obtain the constitution of that parent whom they resemble, hence, of the one who took the leading part in the act of generation. Frequently we find the children of one marriage scrofulous; the father marries a second time, and now begets entirely healthy children; the same takes place sometimes when women marry other men. All that makes generation abnormal favors scrofula; hence, weakness of the parents, in general, and of the sexual capacity, particularly. Thus onanists or fathers who formerly had healthy children, but had sexual intercourse while convalescent from a severe sickness, beget scrofulous children. It seems self-evident, almost, that influences favoring the development of scrofula, generally, if they affect the mother during pregnancy, or while nursing, indirectly carry the disease to the fœtus or infant.

Among these influences belongs also the return of the menses while nursing, or continued nursing during a new pregnancy.

Whether Lalouette is right when he says in his Traité des Scrophules, that the offspring of a conception having taken place during menstruation, comes to the world with scrofula, is questionable without any reliable, comprehensive, and statistic proof.

Even as regards the predisposition of the female sex the views differ.

According to Lepelletier, the scrofulous affections of the female sex compared to those of the male appear in the proportion of 5 to 3; according to Doepp of 4 to 1. Although there is a great distance, no doubt, between the lymphatic temperament, represented by woman, as it were, and the scrofulous state; phthisis, glandular swellings, scirrhous degenerations, in short, diseases in the texture of the tissues mentioned, nevertheless occur oftener in females than in males.

However, let us not be prevented by the above statements from answering the question: wherein consists the essence of scrofula; particularly as most will agree, on closer consideration, that only *one* answer can be given; for we must say: scrofulosis is that dyscrasia which always aims at the formation of purulent exudations. Pyonosos (Vereiterungssucht) we could call it very fittingly, perhaps. There certainly exists, from the very beginning, a wrong proportion in the physiological mixture of the sanguineous elements, similar to that of the rheumatic, syphilitic, and other diatheses; forthwith the power dwelling within every living organism tries to rid it of the defective, pathological blood-elements, though this may refer, pathologically, to the quantitative proportion only between the parts constituting the blood. An excretion takes place, or there appear several peripheric deposits. The contest becomes localized. We witness in this the same centrifugal force which, after an infection with dissecting-poison or variola-poison, at once takes measures to reflect the disease upon the surface. Indeed, the common eruptions of measles and scarlatina, even, may be mentioned as analogies.* The scrofulous localizations, however, are not only characterized by the tendency to puriform decomposition of the exudations produced by a preceding inflammation, but also by the seat itself, *i. e.*, by the preference to certain histological elements, to certain anatomical districts.

Thus it appears to be a most peculiar fact that the local affections of scrofula show themselves with the greatest constancy in the organs of sense; or, more correctly, in their anatomical, auxiliary apparatuses. Scrofulous inflammations of the eyes and ears are the most frequent. The affection of the nose is likewise so well known that one can already diagnosticate the scrofulous habitus from its look. The auxiliary apparatuses of the sense of taste (lips, mucous membrane of the mouth, periosteum—Parulis and Epulis) are also often enough the seat of the dyscrasia. Finally, the most extensive organ of sense, that of feeling, the skin, has undoubtedly to suffer most; it has to intercept as an armor, so to say, the blows which are struck for the radical expulsion of the scrofula-poison. Here, then, the disease relieves itself, the scrofulous cinders being cast out by that Vesuvius, called healthy life-

---

* Even the chronic ulcers of the foot are called by Schroen a reflex of a constitutional disease, against which he recommends Arsenic in alternation with Sulphur. (Hyg., iii, 365–369.)

force, working deeply in the interior, now in the form of aphthæ, now as intertrigo; more unmistakably, it is true, as crusta lactea; ozæna; as blepharitis ciliaris; or, to hold on to the simile, the stream of lava rolls into daylight as the product of an obstinate otorrhœa.

However, we have thus far marked too insufficiently the importance of the lymphatic glandular system in its bearing upon scrofula. Enlarged glands (the maxillary glands, especially) are frequently considered as being identical with "scrofula." These turgescent glands serve, no doubt, as receptacles of the scrofulous elements and products which are directed against and inimical to the normal composition of the blood, and the latter can remain deposited for a time indefinitely long, as does the syphilitic poison in the indurated inguinal canals, until they are brought into course again, as it were, into circulation by a cause more external. From this now results forthwith a localized, new, scrofulous inflammation, with all the terminations possible.

On account of the evident connection of scrofula with the lymphatic (and, very probably, chylific) vessels,* we will direct the attention of the reader to a few physiologico-anatomical facts.

The lymphatic system is an appendix of the venous. The main trunks of the lymphatics run into venous trunks, and smaller lymphatics even are said to open out into veins. The structure of the larger lymphatics agrees with that of the veins in many points. The beginning of the lymphatics is, as yet, not settled beyond dispute. The most popular view is, that the lymphatics originate in certain membranes (*e.g.*, the serous) from closed nets of a much larger diameter than that of the capillary nets of the bloodvessels; while in the connective tissue, on the contrary, they begin with free openings in the interstices of the tissue.

That the lymphatics resorb is sufficiently proven by the reception of the intestinal contents by the chylus-vessels, as well as by the observation that, after ligating the bloodvessels, substances easily resorbable, such as ferrocyanide of

---

* "Of the essence of scrofulosis, Baumgærtner says, we know nothing more reliable than that the lymphatic system, and especially the lymphatic glands, are the principal, and, as it seems, primary seat of the disease."

potassium, for instance, are taken up after some time. But this kind of resorption shows the peculiarity that not all substances are taken up by the lymphatics, and that they require longer time for the process than the bloodvessels. Poisons are usually not taken up by the lymphatics. Hence, after ligating the bloodvessels, an animal cannot be killed by bringing strychnine into a wound of the foot. (Emmert, Henle, Behr.)

This slowness of resorption in the lymphatics is owing, no doubt, to their remaining in the lymphatic glands. On certain and always the same localities of the body (flexor-planes of the joints, interstitial spaces of the muscles, &c.), the lymphatics show a tendency to simplify themselves by a reduction of their numbers. Several of them enter a lymphatic gland to reappear in smaller numbers. The lymphatics, leaving a gland, hunt up now a more distant, second, third, fourth, before they open out into the main lymphatic trunk.

Hence, aside from the chylific system, the lymphatics, as an appendix to the venous system, serve a purpose similar to the former, and the partaking of the lymphatic system in the process of scrofulous affections, allows the deduction that these processes are no strangers to the venous system also. Hence, the genuine scrofulous habitus always shows a preponderance of the venous system also. The typus pasto-venosus is essentially the scrofula-type. Thus we find here guiding-points for a successful therapia, knowing, as we do, a whole series of remedies which have specific relations to the venous constitution.

The function of the lymphatic and lymphatico-glandular system, in their bearing upon the dyscratic morbific matter inimical to the whole economy of life, appears still more plainly, if we quote the simple words of Hyrtl on the relation between the arterio-venous and lymphatico-vascular system.

"The arteries," Hyrtl says, "branch off like trees, by means of countless divisions, into finer and finer branches, which, finally, pass over into veins. The microscopically minute and structureless connecting avenues between the arteries and veins we find in the capillaries. Since the blood streams from the heart into the veins, and from the veins again is brought back to the heart, it makes a circle in its motion, and in so far we speak of a circulation. The capillaries allow certain colorless fluid constituents of the blood to pass through their walls, so as to bring them in contact with the organic particles to be nourished. The organic particles select out of those fluid constituents of the blood, wherewith they are overflooded, whatever they wish to enter into relation with, and want to exchange for the matter used up,—the REMAINDER, LYMPH, returns from those organs through special vessels, called lymphatics, on acccount of their colorless, water-like contents, which open out on certain places into veins. Hence the lymph becomes mixed with the venous blood, and flows back with it to the heart."

A circulation without the co-operation of the lymphatics would be an ideal one. In such a case the organism would have received but suitable (assimilable) material (and everything in normal proportion).

*Scrofulosis, now, manifests itself ab initio as that anomaly of nutrition in which the organic particles, spoken of, are overflooded with so defective a fluid from the capillaries that the lymphatics can scarcely effect the removal of that non-assimilable fluid.*

And whither must this fluid return, finally? From the lymphatics into the veins, from the veins into the heart, from the heart through the aorta, provided the lymphatic glands do not intervene before, again into the surroundings of the organic particles mentioned.

From the excessive activity of the lymphatic system, atonia of the walls, inclosing the lymph, results, for which reason authors of name (Hufeland) pronounced a high degree of atony of the lymphatic system together with a morbidly increased lymph, and a specific dyscrasia thereof, to be the essence of scrofula; its nearest cause. Soemmering seems to have been the first who in scrofulous affections saw a deeply rooted weakness of the vessels of the lymphatic glands, and since Cabanis, Bichat, Pinel, Alibert, Richerand, and most of the contemporaneous writers indorsed this theory it has been generally adopted.

Girtanier attributed scrofula to irritability of the lymphatic system, and it is known that Broussais gave pre-eminence to this theory by all the weight of his name.

Nowhere do we see, hence, the lymphatics work so industriously for our physical welfare as in scrofulosis, and the existence of the numerous lymphatic glands, as mentioned before, no doubt, assist them in their labor. As we have said above, the possibility is afforded by the lymphatic glands for the lymph to become embodied in the circulation after a considerable length of time, only. Indeed, it is certain even, as we have likewise pointed out before, that in the glands the (scrofula) poison (tubercle) may remain inactive for years, encased, as it were, like a mature trichina. "Tuberculosis of the lymphatic glands," Alfred Vogel says, and thus confirms the assertion made, "is not dangerous by itself; tuberculosis of the lungs, however, very usually develops after the appearance of puberty, and this danger must, hence, always be mentioned in our prognosis;" and it is, moreover, not unlikely that the quality of the poison is changed in the lymphatics, perhaps weakened, even, in its intensity of action.

This supposition is based upon the metabolic, change-begetting power of the glands in general. "We are inclined," says Budge, "to accept the cell-formations which appear at the inside of the glandular membrane, and are called enchyma (Purkinje) as the very apparatuses for secretion. We surmise that these cells can assert an attraction, or a change-begetting (metabolic) force upon the liquor sanguinis that courses around them."

Are we to suppose that the inner texture of the lymphatic glands is entirely indifferent as regards the contents coursing through the lymphatics? Scarcely.

The contents of the lymphatics, however, are, without any doubt, of much greater importance than the lymphatics themselves. "From a deficient lymph, arrested in its course," says Baumgærtner, the pathologist already quoted above, who, in this remark of his, squarely hits the nail on the head, "may all the symptoms of scrofula be explained by the phenomena presented to us in the isolated plastic activity, and cellular metamorphosis. If on account of weakness (mostly inherited) of the lymphatic system, a deficient lymph is produced, and arrested in its flow in any part whatsoever, it terminates in isolated plastic activity. Cells are built up therein which, in their turn, attract matter, and thus increase their number, and form tumors. But these isolated cells have a tendency to cellular metamorphosis; they decompose into granula which unite into new cells, pus-cells. By these means the greatest destructions are brought about in all kinds of tissue."

This way of explaining the matter is, in my opinion, based upon a more correct conception than are those other one-sided ideas, according to which the essence of scrofulosis is said to consist, at one time, in a peculiar scrofulous matter (miasma scrofulosum) (Schaefer); at another in an abnormal gastric juice (Willis); now, in acidity of the primæ viæ (Van Helmont); now in an over-amount of albumen in the chylus (Sunderlin); or according to which it is pronounced to be the unfortunate offspring of the monster syphilis, even.

Hausmann, Hecker, Reichelt, Wharton, and Faure assert that the sperma, if not evacuated through the natural channels, is resorbed, and thus produces scrofulous affections; a view which is the crown, so to say, of all theoretical arbitrariness. Hippocrates and Galen attributed scrofula to mucus clinging to the lymphatics, an idea which is based, probably, upon the obtuse guessing that the termination of the dyscrasia in question, as we suppose to-day, has to be searched for in an altered quality of the lymph; though the factor of that change may not have been found out, as yet, beyond dispute; because we cannot, as Baudelocque would have it, declare that the factor to be blamed consists in spoiled air. "If the air," said Baudelocque, "which we inhale, has suffered a change in the relative quantities of the elements constituting it, by a diminution of oxygen or an increase of carbonic acid, hæmatosis necessarily becomes defective and incomplete; and as the blood contains the materials of nutrition and secretion, it must necessarily occasion in the composition of this fluid, alterations more or less harmful, and induce the development of scrofula."

Baudelocque is thus one of the main representatives of the humoral pathology.

With good reason the objection has been made to this theory that, its correctness presupposed, the scrofulous would have to pass through a kind of asphyxia, and would show symptoms accordingly, which, however, is not the case. Besides, in cases of slow asphyxia, the lymphatic glands are never affected. And, then, why should scrofulosis not appear upon the whole globe, provided the conditions for the deprivation of oxygen were present?

*It is more correct, hence, to accuse as ætiological momentum* EVERYTHING *that impoverishes the lymph.* (Borden.)

Hain's view, by the way, is original, which declares scrofula to be a metamorphosis of variola.

The idea indorsed by Ettmueller, Hauter, and others, which, at first sight, lacks both logic and science, and yet does not appear impossible, is that alkalescence OR an acid (which Baumes believes to be phosphoric acid, others a specific one) produces scrofulosis.

But let us abandon now theoretical grounds, and return to the soil of a more correct pathology.

Thus it behooves us to listen to the views of several more recent and famous authors upon scrofula.

## I.

Wunderlich calls scrofula an anomaly of nutrition, whereby, it is true, but little is said.

In advance of it he treats on pimelosis and stearosis, and follows it up by marasmus.*

Wunderlich's statement, according to which scrofulosis is said to have connection with hereditary syphilis, is more important.

Besides coarse, indigestible food, he mentions as other authors do, among the external influences, deficient renewal of air, want of sunlight, upon which causes the fact rests,

---

* He arranges the anomalies of nutrition mentioned (pimelosis, stearosis, scrofula, marasmus), under the head of *autogenetic constitutional diseases*, and counts among them:

*A.* Anæmic forms.

*B.* Plethoric conditions.

*C.* Anomalies of nutrition.

*D.* Hæmorrhagic diathesis.

*E.* Hydrops.

*F.* Constitutional disturbances manifesting themselves by peculiar urinary secretions.

*G.* Rheumatism.

*H.* Gout.

*I.* Constitutional diseases with peculiar multiple localizations.

probably, that the symptoms of scrofula commence during convalescence from other diseases (after measles, hooping-cough, typhus, &c.) Surprising but very pleasing is the confession: "Scrofula characterizes itself, neither by a demonstrable and peculiar change of the blood, nor by products of a peculiar quality."

Almost all parts of the body may show changes, and the anomalies originating are partly hypertrophies, partly serous, plastic, purulent, tuberculous exudations, but very frequently deposits that remain firm; or, thinly purulent, and caseous or ichorous effusions.

The parts especially affected are the lymphatic, secretory and vascular glands, the skin, the subcutaneous connective tissue, the mucous membranes, the brain, lungs, serous membranes, muscles, bones, and joints.

The symptoms may show very different grades.

As regards the habitus scrofulosus, Wunderlich does not differ in his description from the one generally known and accepted.

"This habitus," Wunderlich says, "shows more or less distinctly the lymphatic character; at one time in a certain gross nutrition, accompanied by a thick nose, thick lips, spongy, bloated look, dirty-pale color, coarse and stiff hair, swollen abdomen, thin, and, at the same time, clumsy limbs; at another in a delicate bodily constitution with a thin transparent skin, flushed cheeks, but great sensibility of the parts."

Wunderlich does not mention without purpose, first, the processes upon the skin, then those of the mucous membrane, then those of the lymphatic glands; fourthly, the affections of the bones and joints; and, finally, those of the fatal termination of scrofula,—appearance of tubercles in the brain, the lungs, and other internal parts—thus indorsing, to a certain extent, our theory of the originally centrifugal, and, finally, centripetal direction of the scrofulous anomaly of nutrition.

"The skin of the scrofulous becomes affected by the slightest causes; wounds heal with difficulty, and suppurate for a long time; excoriations secrete and ulcerate; the skin covers itself with obstinate eczematous and impetiginous eruptions, and serpiginous forms frequently appear upon it; the meatus auditorius externus often becomes the seat of an inflammation with purulent discharge.

"In a similar manner the *mucous membranes* are affected; especially, we observe, however, obstinate catarrhs and blennorrhœæ of the eyes, nose, oral cavity, and pharynx; chronic catarrhs of the stomach and intestines, with semi-paralysis (paresis) of the intestinal musculature; catarrhs of the air-passages, often, indeed, with tubercular deposits; catarrhs of the female sexual organs, often with ulcerations; not rarely isolated, local pseudo-growths appear upon the mucosa, which must be considered as a higher development of diseased portions of the mucous membrane.

"The affections most frequent, however, are the swellings and diseases of the lymphatic glands, which show themselves especially in the glands of the throat and neck, but also in the axillary and inguinal, as well as in the bronchial and mesenterial glands, and may appear on account of the most insignificant peripheric affections, and originate spontaneously even. The disturbance therein may consist in hyperæmia, or tuberculous deposits, or hypertrophia.

"Not rarely do we witness among the scrofulous a hypertrophical thickening, and firm infiltrations of single vascular or secretory glands (of the glandula thyreoidea, the ovaries, mammæ, even of the kidneys), mostly with a diminution of their functional capacity.

"As a frequent local manifestation of scrofula, malignant in its nature, we observe affections of the joints, which, at the beginning, show themselves as moderate pathological alterations in the parts surrounding the joints, and are accompanied by swelling and pains. In consequence of frequent relapses and neglect, the evil becomes more stubborn and chronic, the synovial membrane becomes affected, and it may end in firm deposits beneath the latter, or in puriform exudations in the cavity of the joints. Other destructions of the joint may develop therefrom, and the epiphyses may become involved more or less. The affections run a different course in the different joints; at the cervical vertebræ and the knee they lead to induration and swelling, rarely to extensive suppurations; at the joint of the foot they tend toward isolated abscesses and formation of fistulæ; in the elbow-joint to abscesses and fistulæ, which, however, usually heal up, producing anchylosis; in the hip-joint, and at the lumbar vertebræ to the most extensive purulent destructions.

"Next come the affections of the bones, often combined with those of the joints, or existing separately. They may commence at the periosteum, and then terminate either in suppuration, denudation of the bone, or necrosis, or lead to subperiosteal, ossifying exudation; or they start at the bone itself, and appear, at one time, as simple ostitis, and may end in thickening of the bone and hypertrophy, or form purulent products, with the latter of which the construction of new bony substance, in the form of osteophytes or hypertrophical swellings, goes hand in hand, the bones becoming enlarged at times; now and then, however, the affection of the bones is a tuberculous one, to distinguish which from the simple bony ulceration is not possible during life."

The termination in tuberculosis depends (according to Wunderlich) upon the intensity of scrofulosis; it is possible, however, even in case of a scrofulous affection of a lighter grade; while in higher grades, on the other hand, it becomes a necessity, a rule almost.

Tuberculosis may become general; or tuberculous deposits in the mesenterial glands take place; next in the brain and its membranes, in the bronchial glands and lungs.

Finally, ulceration of the bone, congestive abscesses, morbus Brightii, and the development of stearosis, may occasion death.

Even in case of a cure there is inclination to relapses.

Wunderlich's picture of scrofulosis, we see, is sufficiently exhaustive; indeed, in accordance with it, certain histological textures become affected, to which we are usually inclined to attribute a certain immunity, as, for instance, the serous membranes, the mucosa of the stomach, the muscles, kidneys, testicles, ovaries, &c., although we may suppose it as unlikely, *à priori*, that an entire guarantee can be given against scrofulosis with regard to any organ. If we add to this the doctrine of the *pars minoris resistentiæ*, well established, as it is, we may easily explain why now the one individual suffers from the more rare form of a vaginal catarrh, now another from blennorrhœa bronchialis, a third from meningitis (tuberculosa) without the usual initial phenomena of scrofula even.

## II.

As supplements we will quote here now the remarks on scrofulosis of a French writer of high standing, Jousset, though only so far, of course, as he opens to us any new views. (Elements de Médecine pratique, i, 60.)

Jousset names as a characteristic sign of scrofula the deposits of tubercular masses, especially in the lymphatic glands, to which we have given due importance above.

According to Jousset the scrofula-dyscrasia may manifest itself in four forms:

1. As common scrofulosis (forme commune).
2. As malignant (f. maligne).
3. As benignant (f. benigne).
4. As well-fixed, primitive form (f. fixe primitive).

Common scrofulosis comprises the complete development of the disease, thus defining at the same time the fourth form, which does not show either multiple localizations or free intervals, but contents itself with one single attack. It appears in the form of tumor albus, malum Pottii, tuberculosis cerebri, albuminuria, morbus Addisonii, lupus or meningitis basilaris; again as purulent pleuritis and pneumonia, as obstinate inflammation of the eye with destruction of it. Jousset is right in believing that some forms of croup (l'angine couenneuse) must be considered as belonging here, and, above all, phthisis pulmonum.

The designation "fixe primitive" does not preclude the occasional appearance of scrofulous peritonitis, pleuritis, and especially of tuberculous diarrhœa, towards the end of the catastrophe. In the form of common scrofula Jousset distinguishes four periods of development. He confirms what we have already said above, that it belongs to the physiological course, so to speak, that scrofulosis attacks at first the skin, then the mucous membranes (hence, at the commencement, moves in a centrifugal, afterwards in a centripetal direction).

Bazin very adroitly calls the scrofulous cutaneous eruptions scrofulides (who would not think here of syphilides?). These belong either to the moist or dry kind. Among the former, eczema, impetigo (in the face), crusta lactea; among the latter, the erythemata, prurigo, lichen, psoriasis, acne. The swelling of the lymphatic glands in the neighborhood is characteristic of all.

The scrofulous affections of the mucosa comprise that form of coryza accompanied by impetigo of the nasal openings and lips, which finally produce the "mufle scrofuleux;" the obstinate otorrhœa with sero-purulent discharge, "et encore sans carie."

Blepharitis and hordeolum; ophthalmia of still benignant character, granulous pharyngitis with hypertrophy of the tonsils, catarrhal bronchitis, diarrhœa, balanitis, leucorrhœa, and vulvitis among small girls. Scrofulous children are sometimes very fleshy, at others very lean.

Singular as it may seem, Jousset considers rhachitis a disease, strictly to be distinguished in its nature from scrofulosis, and does not agree with the idea (as does Bazin) that the delay in teething, and in learning to walk, is a commencement of scrofulosis, but of rhachitis.

Jousset having acknowledged the systematic progress of scrofula from outward inward (centripetal direction), the second period begins, in his opinion, with the scrofulous affections of the lymphatic glands, and he accepts, in the third only, an affection of the bones and viscera (des viscères), among which we count brain, lungs, pleura, peritoneum, ovaries, liver, pancreas, testicles; regarding panaritia, with caries of the phalanges, a transition state from the second to the third period. Generally a more intense aggravation of the disease, self-evidently, takes place with its progress, and thus the fourth period ends with the developed scrofula-cachexia, of which Jousset gives the following description: "Pale, ash-colored, bloated face, soft, flabby, dry skin; emaciation not too great; serous infiltrations; rarely hectic fever with colliquative sweats, unless there exists, at the same time, phthisis pulmonum. Appetite continues to be good for some time. Colliquative diarrhœa; daily decrease of strength; great indifference. Death from syncope."

One word more on Jousset's malignant and benignant forms of scrofula. He bases the distinction between the two upon the termination in tuberculosis, merely, the latter of which he identifies, without hesitation, with (malignant) scrofulosis. He deems himself justified in so doing upon the following grounds: 1. The scrofulous can beget the tuberculous, and *vice versa.* 2. The tuberculous are often affected in childhood by scrofulous affections (forme benigne). 3. In cases in which the antecedents of the tuberculous show no symptoms of scrofula, the malignant form (*e. g.*, as meningitis tuberculosa), or the well-fixed, primitive form, mentioned above (in the shape of the malum Pottii or tumor albus), may yet make its appearance.

Finally, the chronic character by no means pertains to scrofulosis.

Of the English physicians, Clarke, and of the German, Cannstadt, side with Jousset; who also believe scrofula and tubercles to be one and the same disease. Baumgærtner, on the other hand, remarks: "The forms of the two diseases are very different; therapeutics, frequently triumphant in scrofula, is of no effect in tuberculosis; scrofulous individuals are not much more frequently affected by phthisis than others, and most of the consumptives have had no scrofula at any period of their lives."

The benignant form is said to characterize itself by superficial, local affections, few relapses, and an entire or apparent restitutio ad integrum, even. Females thus affected incline, however, to abortus, dysmenorrhœa, leucorrhœa, and get old early; men cannot stand much, have no endurance, "ne supportent pas la fatigue."

The malignant form, on account of the sudden, simultaneous appearance of the various affections of the gravest grade, is said to remind one of the poisoning by glanders (le farcin). Multiplex abscesses, enormous glandular swellings, sudden carious processes quickly following one another at the most various places of the skeleton; pleuritis of a very acute course, peritonitis, &c., mostly evince, moreover, the malignant character.

Yet in case of a benignant character of scrofulosis, even (forme benigne), the children of those so affected not rarely carry the germ of tubercular meningitis or phthisis within them.

Jousset, aside from the usual momenta (see previous pages), mentions also the following as predisposing: Excessus in venere; pregnancies too often following one another; but especially nursing for too long a time. A stronger predisposition exists likewise after typhus, hooping-cough, and measles.

Bazin calls it a physiological prejudice, that blondes are supposed to have more inclination to scrofula. In his opinion the blonde race is the strongest race, and endowed with most energy. He says that in France just the brunettes and lean, not the plethoric, are affected preponderantly. The French author, who only asserts the frequency of the affection to be equal in Spain, England, and France, no doubt is in error as regards Germany, a country which, in fact, he does not mention, even. He is right, however, in saying that scrofulosis is a disease of the temperate zone. Iceland has no "scrofulous plebs." The torrid zone enjoys the same exemption. The fact is that the disease is much more frequent in wet than dry countries, and, for this reason, is found especially in Holland, Poland, England, Vivarois, in the Sevennes, Alps, Pyrenees, and in gorges and valleys which separate high mountains; besides, it appears that the removal into a cold and wet climate is especially one of the most potent causes of scrofula. Some observers have adduced as illustration that children, who were brought from India to England, became scrofulous there (Buchan, Sam. Cooper). Others have made the same observations with regard to persons who were brought from America and Brazil to France (Guersent). Just as in cold, damp, low, marshy localities, which are deprived of the beneficial influence of air and sun, colorless mushrooms and fungi sprout up, so the scrofulous habitus, under the influence of the same local peculiarities, grows up luxuriantly in numerous specimens without any possibility of arresting it. This cause holds good in the etiology of scrofula as one of the most important and frequent.

## III.

Among the more comprehensive German homœopathic textbooks, Kafka's treatise on scrofula is of prominent interest, especially as he has bestowed the utmost care upon the therapeutic part. We shall return to his experience in this direction, when we speak of the treatment of scrofula. Kafka especially points to the *difficulty of reducing scrofulous exudations.* He considers the process of digestion and assimilation, suffering from a cause not fully discovered thus far (see Baumgærtner), to be the essential terminating point of this dyscrasia. He thinks that in acquired (in contradistinction to hereditary) scrofulosis, the first foundation is already laid in the first few months by overfeeding. Other factors, of no less importance, are want of fresh air and exercise. From these a slow exchange of matter results, and, above all, the necessary processes of oxidation are wanting; hence the prevailing venosity in scrofulosis.

We are reminded, as already mentioned, by those unfortunate and fading creatures, of certain species of plants which are deprived of light and air; pale and bloated, plethoric, not, however, by really healthy juices, but by a watery, colorless liquid, these "miserables" live but half a life. In the same manner, in the animal kingdom, many species of amphibia, with their cold blood and wabbling fleshiness, their construction of limb incapable of quick motion, their indolent, sleepy character, secluded, moisty-cold domiciles, represent scrofulosis with a predominating lymphatic system. This brings us to the ingenious hypothesis of Ruetes on scrofula. He declares the essence of the disease to be a retrogressive metamorphosis, by which the organism attempts to go back to a former stage of life.

Kafka directs our attention to the fact that a too scanty supply of protein-substances favors the development of scrofula. The protein-substances contain, as is well known, Sulphur and Phosphorus. Now, it is remarkable that the two latter frequently are remedies which homœopathists cannot dispense with in scrofulosis.

The authors mentioned above have paid no attention to the closing up of the fontanel at a late date. Kafka especially has marked it out. Even Lepelletier, finally, compares the vital process of the scrofulous with the rapid sprouting (etiolement) of plants deprived of light. Deficiency in the vital functions, poor assimilation, alteration of nutrition, are the necessary consequences of the influences to which most scrofulous individuals have been exposed.

But we must remember, always, that the variety of those influences is great, that for the begetting of what we term scrofula, neither the deprivation of light alone, nor solely the insufficient supply of oxygen, nor a highly non-nitrogenous food, nor one too rich in nitrogen, nor the descent from unhealthy parents suffice.*

On the contrary, a whole series of conditions is wont to show itself as tending toward the development of this disease. Hence it will suffice for us to hold on to the two main factors: the organic predisposition, on one side, and certain disturbances of nutrition contaminating the blood, on the other.

NOTE.—The symptoms of scrofula, it is true, have been divided into local and general. It is difficult, however, to carry out this distinction, since, for instance, the movable swellings in the neighborhood of the lymphatic glands and vessels, which were mentioned among the local, are as well the expression of a constitutional affection, as the degeneration of the bronchial and mesenterical glands (phthisis mesenterica), which are named among the symptoms not purely local. The best proof of the great significance of those swellings, considered to be a purely local symptom, lies in the fact that they are frequently the forerunners of pulmonary tuberculosis, and that two and more children of the same family, at the same time, *i. e.*, when they have attained to a certain age, become invested by such swellings, from which, as mentioned, the ominous tuberculosis results.

In the "Universal Lexicon der practischen Medizin u. Chirurgie" (Leipzig, Voigt and Fernau, 1844), we find a good description of this stadium prodromorum of scrofula; for those swellings ought to be considered as nothing else.

"Most frequently," we read there, "we notice, notwithstanding all the external appearance of health, oviform swellings or globules beneath the skin on places where the lymphatics take their course, and glands are present which, more or less, increase in number, and by and by gain in circumference; at the beginning remain painless for months and years; are fol-

* Though Lugol, even, considers hereditability as the sole cause, and Cullen as nearly the only cause of scrofula; and Lemasson-Delalande says: "It is absolutely impossible that a well-organized being should become scrofulous spontaneously, no matter into what surroundings it might be brought, and be it imprisoned for years, even."

lowed at a later date by heat, redness, local swelling and febrile motions; afterwards fluctuation frequently appears; the skin becomes thinner, ulcerates, and simultaneously or successively allows a substance to penetrate it, resembling the consistency of chestnuts or cheese, or a fluid filled up with purulent or albuminous flakes. The suppuration arising from the lymphatic glands or neighboring tissues, is more or less considerable, and lasts for an indefinite time, amounting to months and even years. At any rate, cicatrization proceeds slowly; the bottom of the ulcers consists of flat or little developed granulation; the edges are bluish-purple, and if they unite, show at the place of the cicatrix, indestructible signs of the disease that has existed; a state of things that arises from the loss of substance of the integuments of the connective tissue of the lymphatic glands, and the agglutinations which the edges of the ulcers form with the muscles beneath the skin. The symptoms usually manifest themselves around the neck, more rarely in the axilla and groin, still more seldom in the fossa poplitea. The skin is, in many cases, the seat of tumors and ulcers, which multiply in various localities of the body. From these ulcers oozes a watery pus, which may leave behind a thick cheese-like (tubercular) mass. During the whole time of this suppuration, likewise lasting for months or years, the edges of the ulcers remain spongy and, some time, muscular surfaces of considerable extent are denuded. In the ratio in which these ulcers increase in number, the general state of health declines; cachexia shows itself; *the disease has become general.*"

---

## DYSCRASIÆ RELATED TO SCROFULA.

### *A.*—TUBERCULOSIS.

We indorse Wunderlich's and Jousset's views, that the tuberculous process appears where the conditions for scrofula have reached their highest degree, and scrofula itself its greatest intensity. When Baumgærtner denies the identity of the two processes on the ground that scrofula does not necessarily terminate in death, while tuberculosis does, we simply reply that the greatest intensity of a disease must needs render the prognosis more unfavorable, and that, moreover, many scrofulous persons die of caries, necrosis, inflammation of the joints, abdominal diseases, exhausting abscesses, &c.

If we compare scrofula with a luxuriantly growing plant, then tuberculosis is the blossom. Now, as there are many plants (*e. g.*, vinca minor; or the so-called porcelain flower, asclepias odorata) which, in many cases, content themselves with a mere luxuriant growth of leaves, so not every scrofulous existence develops its blossom. Or still more correctly, perhaps, the scrofulous affections are the wild offshoots of tuberculosis which, as is well known, seem likewise to be but little adapted to the development of blossom or fruit.

According to Baumgærtner's second objection, most of the tuberculous did not evince any sign of scrofula. This statement is exaggerated, not to mention that, in many cases, the external cause for the development of the scrofulous predisposition existing, may have been wanting, thus far.

If hereditability is assumed as the most evident cause of tuberculosis, we are compelled to concede the same cause to scrofulosis.

And hereditability would much oftener be admitted, were it not that existing tubercles were overlooked, for the reason that they remain stationary, and are harmless in their latent state for any length of time. Thus post-mortem examinations after previous diseases of a non-tuberculous character, have frequently brought to light such tuberculous deposits, *e. g.*, in the apices of the lungs, bronchial glands, &c. *Vice versa*, persons exposed to most unfavorable outside influences did remain free from tuberculosis, since they had no hereditary predisposition to it.

The reason why we cannot make up our mind to refer all such (scrofulous and tuberculous) dyscrasiæ to hereditability, is simply to be found in the fact that modifications of the disease, incalculable in number, are possible which depend upon relations more or less distant from the original individual seat of the infection. However, owing to the fact that herpetic, syphilitic, carcinomatous, chlorotic, and other dyscratic influences are transferred simultaneously, or a surplus of healthy blood from father or mother, asserts its influence during the act of generation, it happens that innumerable varieties and shades of the disease, monoform at the outset, arise.

Thus some members of a family escape with a chronic blepharitis, or an ophthalmia (frequently recurring), or an inclination to bronchial catarrhs, &c., is the only expression of the masked remnant of the dangerous tuberculous inheritance.

Not long ago I saw a child who had the blue eyes of the mother, and the dark-colored iris of the father. If such a differentiation of the parental physical peculiarities were a rule and not an exception rather, we should more frequently meet with pure forms of tuberculosis (and not with bastard forms, *i. e.*, scrofulous affections). Here belongs also that, only exceptionally, the child inherits the blue eyes of the mother and the black hair of the father, and *vice versa.*

### *B.*—Syphilis.

Scrofulosis has often been compared with syphilis, and the former has been considered a masked form of the latter. They resemble each other, it is true, among other things, in this that, in both, the skin so often becomes the seat of the specific deposits; that, moreover, the cutaneous affections (syphilides and scrofulides) in both are apt to be of multiform, or as we are wont to say, polymorph character. But in syphilis the auxiliary apparatuses of the organ of taste (tongue, buccal mucosa) are affected more than in scrofulosis; the ear and eye much less. Except syphilitic iritis there is little mention made of syphilitic affections of the eyes. For the direct infection with gonorrhœal pus (gonorrhœic inflammation of the eyes) cannot be counted here.

The affection of the glandular system would be a tertium comparationis as regards scrofulosis and constitutional syphilitic diseases. Supported by this criterion we could speak of secondary scrofulosis as well as of secondary syphilis. Indeed, the degenerations into necrosis and caries, and the appearance of tuberculosis pulmonum, even, in persons previously scrofulous, might without any arbitrariness be understood as a tertiary phenomenon of the scrofula-dyscrasia. Hufeland divided scrofulosis into *Sc. occulta* and *manifesta.* Syphilidologists cling to this division with regard to syphilis. Even Bazin speaks of masked scrofula.

Even the possibility of transferring the latter by inoculation does not constitute a characteristic distinction between scrofula and syphilis, for although common scrofulosis is not contagious as variola and scarlatina are, nor transferable as is syphilis, vaccinating experiments with pus taken from tubercles have nevertheless given positive results. And how small is the gap between the tuberculous and scrofulous dyscrasia? Moreover, it is a fact, almost, that by transferring the lymph of vaccina-pustules of vaccinated scrofulous children to others, scrofulosis can be communicated to them.

Although it is said that Kortum, Pinel, Alibert, Richerand, Dupuytren, Lepelletier, and others have tried in vain to transfer the disease by laying healthy children into the same bed with scrofulous, or by rubbing, inoculating, or injecting pus of scrofulous children into the skin of healthy ones; yet there exist too many and well-authenticated cases in which children, previously healthy, have been infected by scrofula-dyscrasia since vaccination. Notwithstanding, however, we do not deny that in the surety and certainty with which syphilitic pus causes syphilis, a difference, no doubt, between syphilis and scrofulosis is well established de facto; as scrofulous pus does not, by any means, occasion scrofulosis with the same certainty. Yet we must not forget, on the other hand, that many do not believe secondary and tertiary syphilis capable of being inoculated.

Here belong also the interesting experiments of Sebastian, which have bearing, it is true, upon syphilis only. This Lyonese physician maintains that if we take lymph of a (vaccinated) syphilitic child in such a manner as not to transfer any blood therewith, syphilis cannot be inoculated.* But as soon as the blood of the diseased child gets into the vaccination-wound with the clear, watery lymph, syphilis is transferred (syphilis vaccinalis). Ricord contradicts this view, adducing that: 1. In the clear, watery lymph, even, blood (blood-corpuscles) can be shown to exist microscopically. 2.

* Sebastian, strictly observing his own rules, vaccinated himself with matter of a syphilitic child, and did not become syphilitic.

That it is very difficult so to transfer the blood of one human being to another that it will be resorbed and really become embodied in its circulation. 3. That in view of the frequency of syphilitic affections in large cities, and the difficulty of collecting the poison without any admixture of blood, the number of syphilitic cases transferred by inoculation would be much larger. The second argument adduced by Ricord proves, as every one will see at a glance, just the contrary to that which was to be proven. The very fact that, for the purpose of a lasting embodiment, the blood of one individual as a general thing is difficult to transfer to another, explains the proportionally rare occurrence of an infection by way of vaccination. This holds good with syphilis as well as with scrofulous children. The latter, as I have frequently observed, bleed more copiously on making an incision into the vaccination pustule, and the blood shows a conspicuously dark color (excess of carbon). It is too venous.

As early as 1578 the French Parliament inquired of the medical faculty whether scrofula could be contagious, a question that was answered in the affirmative.

We know now to what extent this answer was erroneous. Certainly no one will assume a real scrofula contagium, such as surely exists with regard to syphilis. For this reason we cannot but agree with Baudelocque, to whom we are indebted for a comprehensive essay upon this subject, and who has proven that scrofula existed several centuries before syphilis, when he argues in the course of his work that the analogies set up between the two diseases are only apparent.

Cullen, Boehmer, Kortum, Gourfand, and others side with Baudelocque; *i. e.*, they also deny such a connection. Kortum in his district had many scrofulous, but almost no syphilitic person, and Baudelocque states that there are a great many syphilitic at Palermo, but almost no scrofulous.

This does not preclude, however, the possibility of syphilitic parents often having scrofulous descendants; yet it happens often enough also, that such children come to the world with syphilitic but not with scrofulous affections. What may have contributed to that error, is the fact, probably, that both diseases, as already mentioned, are apt to have their seat in the same organic parts (skin, lymphatic glands, bones, &c.). We are inclined, however, to find the most positive proof of a relation between the two affections in the fact that the specific remedy against syphilis, mercury (and its various preparations) is able to cure scrofulous diseases innumerable; in short, that the homœopathic antisyphilitica are antiscrofulosa at the same time. Moreover, as mercury in large doses produces the entire picture of the scrofula-cachexia, we must not forget that persons affected by syphilis, who have been fed upon that metallic poison, for this very reason, perhaps, beget children with apparently scrofulous affections. From all this the difficulty is obvious, at least, of defending in a one-sided manner one or the other theory.

### *C.*—Sycosis.

There is another dyscrasia, finally, that has specific relations to the (lymphatic) glandular system, sycosis. An essential mark of the sycotic constitution is, according to Virchow, the excess of white corpuscles in the blood. With good reason v. Grauvogl asks: Whence this excess? The same author quotes in his text-book of homœopathy (§ 297) the following remarks of Autenrieth, bearing on this point: "Sycotic glandular formations appear even in places where otherwise no glands can be found. Thus a degeneration of the glands cannot make up the essence of this disease; the scrofulous glandular swellings, however, always have their seat in the glands originally present." Besides, he points to the difference between sycotic and scrofulous affections of the bones. If the chronic form of sycosis attacks the bony system the affection shows itself in the bones of the nose, buccal cavity, hard palate, superior and inferior maxilla, sternum, os sacrum, ribs, and the processus spinosi. In ozæna sycotica the fetid smell is absent. Upon the whole, the bones are not attacked by sycosis immediately, but the affection starts at the soft parts, or the periosteum; no carious form ever appears, as in syphilis, but only necrosis with formation of sequestrum and sclerosis; and while bony substance destroyed by syphilis, scrofulosis, and tuberculosis is never repaired, a new, dense, bony mass, endeavoring to fill up all the loss occasioned, forms after the cessation of sycotic necrosis. We are of the opinion that criteria, so well marked, fully justify a distinction between scrofulosis, syphilis, and sycosis. However, in view of the confounding chaos which, nevertheless, may be possible, regarding syphilitic, scrofulous, sycotic, psoric, and other dyscratic affections, we have, in my opinion, but one reliable guide. For the Ariadne thread that leads us out of this labyrinth consists in the specific remedy. From the fact that Acid. nitr. cured one case, Iodium another, Sulphur a third, the nature of the disease manifests itself. Here we had before us not only the foundation of a rational therapia, but also of a rational pathology. Let us remember, however, that Hahnemann has laid this foundation. Hence *ex juvantibus*, as we say, we must infer the syphilitic, scrofulous, or any other disease-genus. Thus we should at once have proven the existence of a scrofulous diathesis where Iodium has effected the cure of any morbid process whatsoever. For, among other affections, Iod. cures the indolent infiltrations of the lymphatic glands pathognomonic of scrofula (v. Grauvogl, ii, 210). In this way the riddle is solved, why an obstinate gonorrhœa is suddenly cured by the aid of antipsoric remedies; why, *vice versa*, Iodium and Fer. jodat. are frequently given in vain (for the diagnosis of scrofulosis was a wrong one); why a violent neuralgia disappears without any trace whatever upon the administration of antisycotic remedies; a fact of which Gallavardin has recorded remarkable examples. Then it requires no heroic treatment, no alterative method, no overfeeding with mercury, no Zittmann's cure, either large or small; nay, submissive and gentle as the refractory horse when it has found the right rider; the evil combated so long in vain takes a turn under the influence of the specific remedy.

As regards the course—to mention it by way of explanation—we observe it in scrofulosis to be less fixed than in syphilis, the stability and successive outbreaks of which can be stated more easily and almost predicted. A chancre of the penis will never return the second time, if there has been no new infection; a scrofulous ophthalmia may make relapses, and does, indeed, as a rule return. A scrofulous ozæna maligna may be cured, but the possibility of a return is not excluded.

## *D.*—Rhachitis.

The fact that the same conditions which hasten the development of scrofula occasion rhachitis also, already points to a certain relation between the two. Among those conditions belong, among other things, bad and spoiled air in dwellings. On this account, also, rhachitis progresses most rapidly at the time of spring, while it decreases after the children have exercised in the open air during the summer. In the Southern climate rhachitis does not show itself. The nutrition of the bones is deficient in this disease, and the trouble depends not only upon a want of the salts which might be supplied by importation from without, but the essence of the dyscrasia consists in not assimilating the salts of lime introduced by food. Likewise the bone does not soften in its entire diameter, but at its surface only.

Healthy bones are changed in a threefold manner:

1. By deposits of cartilage-cells upon the periphery.
2. By ossification of these cells.
3. By resorption of the layers looking toward the medullary cavity, a process by which the cavity gradually enlarges.*

Cranium, thorax (ribs), pelvis, and bones of the extremities are most frequently exposed to the rhachitic process.

As in scrofulosis, hereditary influences can frequently be proven. Father and mother usually exhibit, then, the peculiar rhachitic shape of the cranium with very prominent frontal and parietal eminences.

Rhachitis in children of noble birth (in which cases the bad air of dwellings is of less weight as an etiological momentum) can be traced sometimes to a syphilitic affection (though it may have run its course long ago) of the father.

The rhachitic disturbance of nutrition resembles, moreover, the scrofulous in its unexpected appearance during convalescence from diseases of a grave character.

Finally, the results of allopaths with cod-liver oil, and ours with Silic., Calc. carb., Acid. phosph., Phos., &c., point to an essential concordance.

---

* The femur of a child can be placed into the cavity of a full-grown femur, a fact which proves that the infantile femur gradually regenerates itself completely.

## Pathological Anatomy.

Although Wunderlich maintains that the blood of scrofulous persons, and the products of scrofulosis contain nothing characteristic, we must, nevertheless, stop for a moment at the pathological anatomy of this dyscrasia.

Hypertrophy, ulcerations, suppurations, and tubercles result from the scrofulous process. The chronic course is a sufficient characteristic of all. Besides the transition from one into another, *i. e.*, their alternate appearance, is peculiar to them. In place of the eczema or impetigo an ophthalmia may set in, as well as a meningitis in place of lymphatic swellings.

The lymphatic glands especially degenerate hypertrophically; their cellular elements multiply—hyperplasia—a complete resorption is not excluded.

The scrofulous ulcer easily becomes phagedenic, shows itself, aside from its appearance upon the skin, upon the mucous membranes, and frequently produces hypertrophy of the ulcerous tissue.

It exhibits the following character: hard, uneven edges, which are undermined; it is painless, and its surroundings show a pale or violet shiny redness; its bottom is covered with some lymph or thin pus; when it heals, it leaves *ugly*, *deep*, and *hard cicatrices*.

The suppurations generally produce a serous pus with an admixture of caseous elements.

The scrofulous caries exhibits a combination of ulceration and suppuration, which appears in a threefold form:

1. Simple caries.

The bony tissue is infiltrated with blood and atrophies, but the membrana medullaris hypertrophies. The purulent infiltration immediately follows the bloody. From this results a spongious condition of the bone, which softens, ulcerates, and discharges a sanious blackish pus with fragments of bone.

2. Caries with sequestrum, s. pseudo-necrosis, is distinguished from the former by the dying off of a considerable piece of bone, and thus exhibits a transition-form between caries and necrosis.

3. If we find well-marked deposits of tubercle in the bony tissue, we have a third form before us, tuberculous caries.

The tubercular mass is concentrated upon one point, and the bony tissue infiltrated with it. In the latter case there exists simultaneously interstitial hypertrophy, which represents a kind of ivory-ossification, and ends in necrosis.

Spina ventosa appears in the long bones only, and consists in hypertrophy of the membrana medullaris, and a considerable thinning of the bony cylinder. In contradiction to the negative results, which, according to Wunderlich, have issued from the analysis of the blood and pus of scrofulous persons, the pus of scrofulous individuals, according to Gendrin, is said to distinguish itself from that of the non-scrofulous by a larger percentage of soda, and chloride of sodium. Preuss ascribes to it caseine such as belongs to the tubercle. Finally it is asserted, that the urine shows oxalic and uro-benzoic acids in considerable quantities.

In persons who have died of scrofulosis, we find the indurated glands changed into a whitish-gray, more or less fatty, and often almost cartilaginous mass; in some cases they have changed into the caseous mass which also appears in the pulmonary tubercle, the caseous substance being frequently softened in the centre and transformed into pus.

However, let us turn as early as this, even, to the essential part of our task, which consists in framing in the special pictures of scrofulosis, in which the remedies soon to be mentioned find their place, as well as in giving special and precise indications for the several antiscrofulosa, and in proving their efficacy by clinical examples.

# II.

# THE SPECIAL FORMS OF SCROFULA.

## *A.*—The Cutaneous System.

The skin, Wunderlich says very truly, is the most sensitive organ for constitutional disturbances, and in none of them remains entirely intact. The anomalies of the skin, brought about by the co-operation of scrofulous constitutional disturbances, appear polymorph with forms well marked but little characteristic. It is always as difficult as important a task to recognize, aside from the local changes, the constitutional disease lying at the bottom.

The scrofulous cutaneous affections do not belong either among the cutaneous neuroses, or the independent cutaneous hyperæmiæ;—(roseola, erythemata, erysipelas-forms) or the anomalies of cutaneous secretions—sudori-sebaceous secretions*—or among the hemorrhages or apoplexies of the skin, but may be arranged most properly among the exudations. These exudative processes upon the skin show very manifold forms, which depend partly upon the nature of the product, partly upon the character of the parts principally affected, but are inexplainable for the most part. They appear in a fourfold form:

1. As noduli, papulæ—strophulus; lichen; prurigo.
2. As hives (pomphi; urticaria).
3. As serous exudations beneath the epidermis—vesiculæ and bullæ—eczematous forms—miliaria—herpetic forms—rhypia.

---

* The hordeolum (stye) so frequent among the scrofulous constitutes an exception.

4. As elevations of the epidermis filled with lymph or pus; as pustules—impetigo, acne-pustules—ecthyma.

Only the two latter exudative forms are of interest to us, here, they being truly characteristic of scrofulosis.

The process in the development of the eczematous form is the following:

Upon a portion of the skin, more or less hyperæmic, small vesicles appear, which mostly stand closely together, have watery clear or wheyish contents, and cover a surface indefinite in form and extent. The eruption is generally accompanied by stinging and burning.

The vesicles terminate—

Either by bursting, and lamellose desquamation of the epidermis;

Or by the formation of crusts, more or less thick;

Or they become chronic by successive eruptions, and thus occasion a change of the skin, which exhibits intensely chronic injections, deposits a very thin epidermis, never attaining to any degree of density, and shows great inclination to serous secretions. The metamorphosis of the vesicles, last mentioned, exactly corresponds to the scrofulous eczema. This eczema has also been termed *eczema rubrum* (in contradistinction to E. simplex and E. chronicum). However, it always exhibits a form which, developing with intense hyperæmia and corresponding violent burning, frequent and considerable swelling of the subcutaneous cellular tissue and fever, mostly befalls the face. The vesicles, having turbid contents, burst, and the cutaneous surface appears abraded. This form frequently becomes chronic on account of fresh eruptions.

The eczema of the cheeks may also be designated as E. rubrum, which, on account of its antagonistic relation to the uropoetic apparatus, we have mentioned above.

However, since genuine eczema does not occur very frequently in scrofulosis, but, in most cases, shows itself in combination with serous and purulent exudations; the forms accompanied by pustular developments are not of any less interest to us, and among these again the impetiginous eruptions especially.

They consist in small pus-vesicles, which appear in irregular clusters upon a surface more or less hyperæmic; soon burst and, by means of their contents, and in consequence of a continuous exudation, form flat, thick, firm or friable crusts.

Sometimes they run through their course rapidly, and heal up in from three to four weeks; mostly, however, they drag out for a greater length of time, and become very chronic by successive eruptions or slow growth of the crusts.

As concomitants we observe sometimes fever during the eruptive stage, and frequently swelling of the *neighboring lymphatic glands.*

As we have already pointed out, the exudative form, consisting of impetigo and eczema—eczema impetiginodes, impetigo eczematodes—is, no doubt, the most frequent, though we must also mention the genuine forms:

*Impetigo erysipelatodes* with prominent hyperæmia; located in the face, especially.

*Impetigo figurata;* round or oval form of the eruption (generally appearing in several groups) and of the crusts afterwards formed, which occasionally become confluent. The latter frequently have a honey-like appearance (melitagra). They are found mostly in the face, also at the upper extremities of young persons, and run an acute or subacute course.

*Impetigo larvalis*, especially among children; a chronic form with confluent crusts of a brown color, or a color changed by the admixture of dirt. They cover the face like a mask (crusta lactea; tinea mucosa; achores).

The MILK-CRUST—CRUSTA LACTEA—is probably always associated with scrofulosis. This eruption, as is well known, disfigures children considerably. They scratch it, knock against it, and thus occasion is given for discharge of blood, and painful and too early detachment of the crusts. The surroundings of the eyes often participate in the affection, so much so, as to make the latter appear crusted over, almost; though two blue, unharmed pupils may generally be seen through the opening left. The tender skin is turgescent, and upon laying the hand upon the inflamed spots of the head and face, a burning heat is often felt.

This form of impetigo is not hard to cure, but its sudden disappearance is frequently followed by the most dangerous consequences to the health and life of the child. Such a sudden drying off of the eruption I have observed after

Silicea (if the eruption appeared on the head), followed by a real withering of the children who, but a short time before, were fleshy, and showed no signs of suffering from disease. For this reason the dose of the proper remedy ought not to be repeated too often.* The worst consequences, however, result from the brusque besmearing and drying out of the eruption by means of lead or zinc salves, and even from the external application of cod-liver oil, which ought not to be thought of here.

On account of such attempts at cure a sudden transposition of scrofulosis to inner organs may happen, no doubt; a fatal pneumonia, meningitis, general marasmus, without any visible local disease even, may result. However, those disinclined to believe Hahnemann in this respect, will probably believe Hufeland, who says: "We must always try to direct the disease toward the outer parts; cutaneous eruptions we ought not to attempt to cure." Hufeland, of course, had reference to old-fashioned allopathic attempts at cure.

Wunderlich mentions an *impetigo scabiosa;* an extensive, very thick, bark-like formation of crusts, frequently spreading over a whole limb with sanious secretion, and often with ulceration. I observed this form to run across the face: hard, dry, now elongated, now round, elevated crusts, more disseminated, and well marked off from the healthy parts.

Very often the auricula is affected by such impetiginous eczemata, especially in case of simultaneous otorrhœa. But they appear at the neck and arms, even. *Calcar. carb.* in alternation with *Lycopod.* is specific. Now and then *Ferrum jodat. sachar.* hastens the cure in a remarkable manner.

*Impetigo decalvans*, with sure loss of the hair. (*Graphit.* 30; *Arsenic* 9–24.)

*Impetigo granulata:* Scattered groups of crusts upon the hairy parts of the head. (*Silic.*, *Mercur. viv.* 3d triturat.)

*Impetigo sparsa:* Scattered small groups of pustules which may be found on different parts of the body (obstinate). (*Arsenic.*)

---

* Next to Silic., Calcar. is to be considered, especially if the children are pale, and suffer from habitual diarrhœa. Sulphur in case of a large abdomen and constipation.

*Impetigo rodens:* Phagedenic, enlarging ulcers, covered with crusts which, however, very rarely occasion any loss of tissue in depth. (*Kal. jod.*)

More frequent and, hence, more characteristic of scrofulosis than most of the impetiginous eruptions last mentioned is

*Blepharitis ciliaris,*

which rightfully finds its place here.

The inference as to a relation existing between the two is already justified for the two reasons that Silic. is just as efficacious against blepharitis as it is against those impetigo-forms upon the hairy portion of the head, and that, moreover, scrofulous persons are affected by *both* diseases so exceedingly often; inflammation and deposits of a plastic exudation into the connective tissue surrounding the glands of the hair-bulb are, likewise not absent, and the crumbling, friable, dirty-colored masses agglutinating the ciliæ distinguish themselves in nothing from the product of genuine impetiginous eruptions. However, homœopaths need not ask with anxious care, whether this form more deserves the name of impetigo *figurata*, or that should be called *larvalis*, &c., rather. Such a pedantic classification would be of profit only if a fruitful therapia could be based thereupon. But the latter is very rarely the case with professional dermatologists. As regards the contradistinction between homœopathy and those gentlemen, we may say, perhaps, that it resembles that between Jussieu's and Linné's system. We do not care any for the artificial nosological name which was obtained only by starting from this or that arbitrary principle of classification, but we do care, above all, for the *natural* relation of the several diseases among themselves; we search for the complexes of disease-phenomena, and compare them with similar complexes or pathological pictures. Thus the local reflexes of scrofulosis are to us but points of support, hints and guides for remedies, more or less universal, eradicating the evil.* The concomitants of the scrofulous exanthema are considered, at the same

* For: "Les lesions de texture sont la manifestation anatomique et sensible de la maladie; mais la maladie dans son essence et son point de départ est toute dynamique."

time, and have an influence upon the selection of the remedy, often more decisive than the anatomical region of the eruption. The slaves of nomenclature never were great therapeutists.

We will yet mention that ophthalmologists speak of a *crusta lactea palpebrarum*. This eczema of the lids appears by itself, or in company with facial eczema. The small vesicles filled with a yellowish liquid burst, the secretion excoriating the neighboring parts; crusts are forming, and frequently the entire lid appears to be one ulcerated surface. From the complications of this palpebral eczema which may possibly occur together with blepharitis ciliaris, inflammation of the lid-glands, the close connection of these eruptive diseases with the scrofula diathesis is plainly evident.

For this very reason we will interpone at this place the description of this frequent scrofulous localization, *i. e.*, of blepharitis ciliaris, and not where we speak of the affections of the glandular system or eye.

The common inflammation of the glands of the hair-bulbs of the lids, blepharitis, more corectly blepharadenitis ciliaris, is said to affect the upper lid most frequently, is mostly bilateral and characterized by redness, swelling, and inclination to punctiform abscesses in the edge of the lid. The edges of the lids, on account of the plastic exudation deposited into the connective tissue surrounding the glands, assume a tuberous, knotty shape and firmness. At the beginning, fine scales, dependent upon an increased secretion of the glands, show themselves around the basis of the several ciliæ which may be observed as surrounding the latter in ring-form, and when detached, as adhering to them in the form of circular scales. After the detachment the bottom around the cilia is slightly excoriated and even bloody, and encircled by very minute vessels. If no resorption takes place, the edges agglutinate during the night and photophobia sets in, which grows more and more intense; the eyes tire out by working at things near. Now commences the formation of abscesses not in the glands of the hair-bulbs, but in the connective tissue enveloping them; the hair-bulbs remain intact until displaced by oft-recurring inflammation, suppuration and cicatrization of their glands and the adjacent tissue; they are deprived of nutrition, degenerate, decay, and are cast off. Thus originates *trichiasis madarosis* and, by subsequent deposits of plastic or indurating exudations, *tylosis;* in the lower lid, *ectropium.* Hyperæmia of the conjunctiva palpebrarum and blepharospasm accompany the more profuse secretion of the mucous follicles and Meibomian glands; the tears, secreted more copiously now, corrode the sore places freed from the crusts; the tears being collected behind the ectropic and hypertrophic lower lid, make the eye appear as if it were swimming in water; the puncta lacrymalia close up, or located more outwardly, do not extend any longer into the lacus lacrymarum, and the tears flow over the cheeks (*epiphora*). At a later date tarsomalacia and deformities of the cartilages, ectropium and epidermoid degeneration of the conjunctiva of the lids appear as complications of the former.

Another complication consists in the so-called *asthenopia—decrease of energy in the ciliary nerves of the eye*—Romberg—anæsthesia with subsequent optic hyperæsthesia, which requires the use of blue spectacles. According to Begin, intent looking, when doing fine work, is said to be the ætiological momentum of it.*

Aside from the glands of the hair-bulbs of the lids, the sebaceous glands of the lids are extremely often affected in scrofulosis, from which the well-known styes — (hordeola) originate. The hordeolum is neither a furuncle (since it does not discharge a cord and leaves no cicatrix), nor an inflammation of the Meibomian glands (Desmarres, Juengken), nor of the glands of the hair-bulb mentioned before (Leis). The hordeolum has nothing to do, moreover, with the *chalazion* (a tumor seated in the cartilage of the lid), or the *milium*, a nodulus originating in the sebaceous glands of the skin. We give these researches of more recent observers more for the sake of completeness, than for the reason that the nice discussion upon the essence of the various processes in the lid will be of any influence upon our therapeutics. For, aside from the fact that several of the affections named may be present

* The author experienced on himself that even after protracted reading of small type—a number of the Berliner Volkszeitung—at dusk, a complete hordeolum developed within a few hours. To the subjective predisposition an objective cause must apparently always correspond.

simultaneously, and, according to experience, often are present; it must suffice for us to know whether a suppurative process is to be expected or not, and to this our therapeutic attention directs itself. Whether the sebaceous, Meibomian, or hair-bulb glands, are the seat of the abscess, &c., is evidently of but little importance; for, upon the strength of this one fact we should not be able to prefer *Mercur.* to *Silic.*, or any other remedy, hastening the suppurative process, to *Hepar.* Other indications determine the selection of these several remedies. As a rule, the common stye always heals under the administration of SIL. (6–30) from one to two doses daily, according to the acute character of the case.

Next, the cutaneous tubercle comes up for consideration. It consists in infiltrations of the cutis which owe their origin mainly to scrofulous constitutional anomalies—disturbances in the return of the blood and lymph. Mechanical, local injuries, are sometimes the cause of the formation of such cutaneous infiltrations. The spot is mostly elevated, of a red or brown color, circumscribed and resistant.

Cutaneous tubercles heal with difficulty by resolution, frequently under exfoliations, and with subsequent cicatrix-like contractions, or after previous softening and formation of pustules; but they often persist for years, and may give rise to superficial or deeper ulcerations. The several forms to be distinguished are:

1. Acne-tubercle (acne rosacea, mentagra).

2. Lupus, located most frequently in the face, especially on the nose and cheeks. Both do not belong among the characteristic, scrofulous eruptions. Of the lupus-forms, probably the one described as lupus *elevatus non exedens* does. The noduli appear here above the level of the skin in groups as elevations of the size of a lentil, are flattened, and, at a later period, become confluent, and show a yellow, red or reddish-brown color. They are of moderate consistency, gradually form plateaus or wall-like elevations from $\frac{1}{2}'''$ to $2'''$ in height, which, however, are furrowed by incisions; the epidermis detaches itself upon their surface, yet becomes more and more dense, scaly, even crusty, especially if some of the spots are discharging. The affection spreads by new groups

of tubercles at the periphery, while the older remain as they are, or sink in and dry up, forming cicatrices.

Among the remedies against acne-tubercle (especially against mentagra) as well as against the lupus-forms, *Arsenic.* and *Caustic.* deserve the greatest confidence, *Clematis* against simple acne, papulæ, and sycosis.

Next to the cutaneous tubercle come the deep suppurations of the skin, standing midways, so to say, between the pustular forms and the infiltrations of the cutis. As principal representation of the deep suppuration of the skin,

*The Boil—Furunculus,*

may be named. It plays a decidedly double role in scrofulosis. It appears sporadically, *i. e.*, at shorter or longer intervals separate boils develop, which signify that something in nutrition is at fault, be it called a humor or miasma scrofulosum, or by any other name whatsoever; in short, the furuncle most surely carries away certain cinders of the blood, or something else not beneficial to the entire economy; or (in view of the same aim) a rising *en masse* of boils, so to say, takes place. We could call them a monster demonstration of scrofulosis. The whole body is covered with boils more or less. The critical nature of this eruption is to be doubted still less; for it is preceded by a general decline, dependent, as it seems, upon scrofulosis of the mesenterial glands. After emaciation, increasing to a skeleton-like appearance with aged look, has preceded for weeks, nutrition is entirely prostrated, and atrophy has reached its highest degree; the organism still succeeds sometimes in producing a restitution of the inner organs by the development of those furunculous inflammations *en masse*. Aside from genuine boils, knotty abscesses, especially beneath the scalp, with a sympathetic affection of the swollen lymphatic glands, are not a very rare phenomenon, and undoubtedly of a purely critical nature. We always succeed with *Silic.* in maturing the single boil, the breaking of which may be preceded by violent pains and chills. If the treatment of the multiple furuncle takes place after a grave internal disease, *Sulph.* 30 is preferable, or indicated, at least, after *Sil.*

If the boil is located at the upper eyelid, the latter is frequently attacked by phlegmonous inflammation, and the pains reach the highest degree. Discolored, livid look, firm swelling, often as hard as a board, and fever. Here *Mercur. sol.* and *Acid. nitr.* are well indicated after *Bellad.* In case of threatening gangrenous decomposition, *Arsenic* (*Apis*, *Carb. veg.*, *Laches.*).

The course of boils, upon the whole, is too well known to spend a single word on it. *The exudation, consisting of a lump of coagulated fibrin* (cord), which is mixed with fragments of tissue, and pervaded and covered with blood- and pus-corpuscles, is essential. The cord, at the beginning still intimately connected with the adjacent tissue-parts, becomes detached by progressive suppuration; simultaneously the swelling increases still more, the upper layers of the skin are consumed and break, and, on moderate pressure, the cord-like mass together with a bloody pus, is evacuated *in toto*, leaving a cavity which closes up within a very short time with a small punctiform cicatrix.

Very often, however, a general abscess develops from the original furunculous inflammation, the breaking of which is preceded by distinct fluctuation, a circumstance under which the characteristic appearance of the cord cannot be reckoned upon.

But few affections of the cutis and its appurtenances, preponderantly belonging to scrofulosis, remain for discussion now.

### *Intertrigo.*

The detachment of too young an epidermis, on places where the skin forms folds and recesses, can scarcely be attributed always to uncleanliness and fleshiness, especially as the secreted smeary-mucous, often incrusted, now and then seropurulent or offensive mass, as well as the obstinacy of the affection in single cases, and its extension with general fiery redness of the skin, sufficiently point to the specific significance of the trouble. Intertrigo will hardly ever owe its origin to simply mechanical conditions; against this argues, on the one hand, its appearance upon one side only (*e. g.*, under one arm), and its transition into other, for instance, herpetic exanthemata.

This shows the irrationality of treating, or driving away intertrigo, with exsiccating salves or powders, such as Lycopod-powder, starch-powder, &c., which answer the same purpose.

On the other hand, *Lycopod.*, in a homœopathic preparation, given internally, has proved its efficacy, we may say, perhaps, in a very singular manner. Yet where it has already been used externally, we must give *Sulph.*, or another remedy corresponding to the complications of the trouble.

Next to intertrigo come the species of *pityriasis*, which, in a strict anatomical view, likewise represent an anomaly in the formation of the epidermis which may be referred to a disturbance of nutrition.

Since the connection between pityriasis and scrofula appears to be less evident than that of intertrigo, we pass on, at once, to

### *Psoriasis.*

In districts (cities) where scrofula is endemic, as it were, children are brought to us now and then, who are affected over the whole body with a scaly eruption. The epidermical lamellæ, which can be detached very easily, lay upon a reddened bottom. Many spots, on account of their easy bleeding and watery discharge, remind one of eczema or impetigo, though they must not be counted among them. The possibility of a sudden spreading of the exanthema, its power for luxuriant growth, and the want of preference for certain localities, are characteristic of it. On the contrary, psoriasis, leaps or creeps hither or thither, occupies the face as well as the lower extremities, abdomen, calves, &c. It seems incomprehensible, how authors of name, on the one hand, admit of a hereditary predisposition to psoriasis, on the other, attempt to refer its existence to local causes (with bakers, storekeepers, &c.) to taking cold, the use of highly seasoned food, and then again to depressing affections of the brain.

We need not stop at the origin of the several species of psoriasis from small, round, disseminate, rose-red spots, &c. We take the picture in its full development, and point out that to psoriasis of the scrofulous—and this only interests us here—*Arsenic.* most frequently corresponds homœopathically; next *Graphit.* (hence the specifics against eczema rubrum), and *Causticum.*

We have no right to treat of scabies here, since it appears wherever the acarus has access; we will, however, not omit the remark, that dyscratic, hence scrofulous individuals, even, are more exposed to the influence of the acarus, and are visited by more obstinate consequences than healthy persons. Besides, we direct the attention to our remarks in our treatise on Sulphur as a remedy against scrofulous diseases.

### *Favus—Tinea favosa.*

Favus, considered though it is by many dermatologists as solely depending upon vegetable parasites, just as plica polonica is declared by the most short-sighted natural philosophers to be but a local disease of the scalp, may certainly be looked upon more correctly as the expression of a scrofulous constitution. Cazenave is very right in asking the question: "If the disease were a formation of microscopical fungi, how, then, can favus disappear so suddenly during the course of pleuritis or typhus? Besides, how can a favus pustule around a hair give rise to other pustules in places where no hairs are to be found?" If the hair is not essentially necessary to this evil, why does the contagious favus not always spread over the skin more and more? (Prag. Viertelj. 5, Jahrg. iv, s. 59.)

Favus, in its fully developed form, presents a crust of grayish-yellow color, round shape, and mealy consistency, which is depressed in the centre, confluent, almost pustular without containing any pus, however, and has a smell resembling that of the urine of cats. Each crust is built up from a countless number of fungous bodies and fibrils.

These formations are inhabited not unfrequently by lice, occasion other eruptions, excoriations, and ulcerations, ruin the hair, and produce infiltrations into the lymphatic glands of the neck.

If we add that such patients grow dull gradually, and their mental development stands still, we have reason to rejoice over the fact that homœopathic literature, at least, can show reliable and real cures, while the allopathic school confines itself merely to mechanico-surgical assistance.

Let us briefly recapitulate the therapia of scrofulous cutaneous diseases, in order to make some additions by way of complement. "We ought to make no attempt at healing eruptive diseases." In these words of the ingenious Hufeland, already quoted above, the danger which an *external* treatment of scrofulous cutaneous affections would have in its trail, is hinted at. We homœopaths do not abandon, however, a specific internal treatment. Our curative apparatus is exceedingly simple, notwithstanding; we pay principal attention to the locality of the eruption, and to its dry or serous or purulent character. Thus *Arsenic.* corresponds in most cases to the scrofulous eczema (E. rubr.). Two drops of the sixth or second dilution in twelve teaspoonfuls of water, a teaspoonful morning and evening, suffice. In case of simultaneous obstruction, and when the hairy scalp is affected, at the same time, *Mercur.*, *Silic.*, and *Graphit.* (the eruption behind the ear being characteristic of the latter remedy).

*Ferrum jodat.* is required generally at the close of the cure. If the intensely itching spots bleed easily, *Nitr. ac.* is preferable to *Arsen.*

Eczema impetiginodes (eczema with purulent discharge) requires *Hep. sulph. calc.*, the characteristic indications of which Hirschel enumerates in the interesting case of LVII, or *Calc. carb.*, if the face is attacked (XXXIX), or *Mercur.*, if the hairy scalp presents one purulent surface almost (LXXXVI). Besides Hep. sulph. calc.; *Sulphur* claims the same importance (CXII and CXXVII). Even if the cure requires weeks, the remedies mentioned nevertheless deserve more confidence than the vegetable drugs, among which *Viola tricolor* enjoys the reputation of a specific against Crusta lactea (CXXXIII). The same remedies come up for consideration in blepharitis ciliaris, characteristic on account of its frequency among the scrofulous. Here, however, *Silic.* most surely deserves preference to ARSENIC, so important in the most obstinate eczematous eruptions. On the other hand, besides *Silic.; Hepar. sulph. calc.*, as well as *Merc.*, are indispensable in many cases. In complications with styes (suppuration of one or more sebaceous glands of the lid), *Sil.* is likewise in place, to mature the small abscesses. *Graphit.*, in case of intense photophobia, sensation of heaviness of the lids, and itching of the edges. *Graphit.*, moreover, removes the predisposition to styes.

Mention has already been made of the therapia of the cutaneous tubercle (*Arsen.*, *Caust.*, besides *Silic.*, sometimes entirely corresponding to facial eruptions in general, CI), and thus we proceed to the deep suppurations of the cutaneous integuments, so frequent in the life of scrofulous individuals. These suppurations appear in an isolated form as furunculus or carbunculus. The expulsion of the characteristic fibrinous exudation (cord), or the hastening of the abscess (at the spot of the original boil), again is brought about best by *Silic.; Sulph.* or *Mercur.* suits better for certain individualities. A comparison between the pathogenesis of these minerals related in their action, presents the more minute differences. SILIC. seems to correspond more to mature age (to scrofulosis and arthritis), HEPAR to childhood alone (genuine scrofulosis), MERCUR., probably, to scrofulosis upon an originally syphilitic bottom. These criteria regarding the administration of these suppurative remedies mentioned, would apply then not only to blepharitis ciliaris, but also to all other cases. We will, however, not anticipate.

One word more only as regards *Rhus. Rhus toxic.* produces a pure form of eczema, and has proved itself a remedy, especially for that form of it appearing at the nape of the neck. A complication of scrofula with rheuma would, moreover, direct the selection to *Rhus.* The same holds good of *Caustic.*, to which the purulent crusty forms of eruptions correspond.

In tinea favosa which we mentioned lastly, *Arsenic*, with its faculty of destroying parasitic life, deserves consideration. Compare extracts taken from its pathogenesis. Finally, we will mention *cod-liver oil* which, according to Kafka, is indicated in all scrofulous skin diseases, combined with exudations, hence, in eczema, impetigo, &c.

It cannot be too strongly impressed that *one* remedy does not always correspond to the entire morbid state. If we believe, however, that our selection has been a correct one, it is better to change the dose than the remedy. Moreover, in the fact that the cure does not always succeed with *one* remedy, the reason is to be found, why certain remedies marked out as antiscrofulosa, are represented by but few cases, comparatively. For reports, clinical observations with one remedy only, are suitable.

### *B.*—The Muco-Membranous System.

The mucous lining of the organs of sense, of the eye, ear, nose, and mouth, is predominantly affected. Simultaneously a secretion takes place of so acrid a nature as regularly to occasion the development of an eczematous eruption in the neighboring locality. Thus the catarrh of the nasal mucosa produces an eczema in the surroundings of the nasal openings and upper lip, that of the meat. audit. ext. an eczema on the lobe of the ear or its surroundings; that of the conjunctiva, an eczema of the cheeks; that of the gums, an eczema of the corners of the mouth or the chin, but also that of the intestinal tract, soreness of the anus.

The traditional antiscrofulous cures which began with a purification of the primæ viæ (Hufeland) probably owe their origin to this fact. It was believed, *a tout prix*, that too much acidity, or too much mucus was the cause of scrofulosis.

Aside from the mucous lining of the anatomical auxiliary apparatuses of the organs of sense, the mucosa of the air-passages, tractus intestinalis, and genital organs is affected. In these affections we must not lose sight entirely of the principal special forms. At first we will speak, however, of the organs of sense.

## I. ORGANS OF SENSE.

### 1. *Scrofulous Inflammation of the Eye.*

#### (*a.*) COMMON SCROFULOUS OPHTHALMIA.

There is hardly a disease which, in its appearance and course, is so well fixed and conservative as scrofulous ophthalmia. For this reason it can be recognized at a glance, and needs no elaborate diagnosis. Who would not remember that children, thus affected, anxiously avoid the light, spasmodically close the lids, and, when yielding to the friendly persuasion of the physician, are able to open the eyes only with a simultaneous discharge of acrid, corrosive tears. Agglutination of the lids, redness, intense vascular injection of the eye, formation of pustules (the disease being called, therefore, pustular ophthalmia) do not fail to appear. Mostly we observe an unclean complexion, thick nose, blonde hair, and other signs of a scrofulous habitus. Besides, the affection has a great tendency to relapses. Under improper treatment it may drag out for months. Some children, notwithstanding the existing spasm of the lids and the intense photophobia, attain to a certain dexterity in recognizing objects of their surroundings by winking. Others squat for days in corners, and become almost brutalized, giving way, as they do, to the incontrollable desire of searching for dark localities.

It is not practical, although ophthalmologists do so, to separate scrofulous conjunctivitis from keratitis. They appear too often simultaneously, too frequently run into each other, and together form that scrofulous ophthalmia so common nowadays.

If the conjunctiva is attacked, the affection locates mostly in the conjunctiva scleroticæ, not far from the edge of the cornea, around which the exanthema often appears in the shape of a rosary. There appears at first a circumscribed, dense, vascular injection, in the centre of which almost always a plastic exudation, resembling now a pustule, now a nodulus, may be observed at an early hour, and toward which a ramification of vessels of triangular form, with the basis looking toward the orbita, develops itself sooner or later ("scrofulo-vascular ribbon"). If the exudation is deposited very superficially, it is soon discharged in an outward direction, leaving, however, superficial ulcers of small size and unclean appearance; if the exudation is situated deeper, the ulcer becomes deeper and more obstinate. If the exudation is deposited evenly over the cornea, it does not break so easily, and is more apt to occasion *pannus scrofulosus*.

It suffices to remark that the origin of the vesicles is nearly the same in scrofulous keratitis. A reddened spot in the cornea, the vessels of which communicate with those of the conjunctiva, and in which a few days afterwards a vesicle of a dirty-grayish color, as large as a millet-seed, develops itself, above which the epitelium appears to be loosened, shows itself now, and is accompanied by photophobia, more or less intense, discharge of tears, and injection of the conjunctiva. If there is but one vesicle present, it is apt, by depositing a greater quantity of plastic exudation, to enlarge to the size of a hemp-seed, which appears clear at first, but later becomes cloudy and thickish, and breaks sooner or later according to its being imbedded more superficially or deeply. If the epitelium only had to be perforated, a clean superficial ulcer forms with an inclination to heal up soon and completely. If the exudation is deposited more deeply, however, a dirty-grayish ulcer is produced, in the lardaceous edge and bottom of which a fine ramification of vessels may be observed by aid of a magnifying glass. In case of a favorable course, these ulcers may heal very well, but if the disease has progressed so far, as not only to crowd the fibrils of the cornea out of their position, but also to destroy them, the cure succeeds only under the formation of cicatrix-tissue which occasions a lasting opacity. If the ulcers remain for some time in the state of purulent secretion, they not only increase in width, but also in depth. As consequences we observe, then, partial softening and pouching out of the cornea by the contents of the eye-chamber (*keratoconus*), or perforation and its results; discharge of the liquid of the eye-chamber, prolapse of the iris, &c.

The latter eventualities have to be marked out, especially in order to place in proper light the value of homœopathic treatment, so specific against scrofulo-pustular ophthalmia.

The following we quote from Dr. Boyer's prize essay: "On Scrofulous, Herpetic, and Rheumatic Ophthalmia, and their Homœopathic Treatment."

Prof. Velpeau sees in every scrofulous inflammation a simple one only; according to Boyer, however, the three kinds of ophthalmia have only the chronic course (in Hahnemann's sense, s. Organon, § 78) in common.*

### *Scrofulous Ophthalmia*

Boyer divides into:

1. *Genuine Scrofulous Ophthalmia*, which shows itself either as conjunctivitis scrofulosa or as scrofulous sclerotitis (termed also scrofulo-rheumatic, *i. e.*, a kind of conjunctivitis attacking both sclerotica and cornea).

---

* According to Mackenzie, ninety out of a hundred cases of ophthalmia of children are scrofulous ophthalmia, and this well-marked and characteristic disease is not seldom the first manifestation of scrofulosis.

2. *Non-vascular, Primitive Keratitis.*

3. *Scrofulous Blepharo-adenitis.*

TERMINATIONS OF SCROFULOUS OPHTHALMIA.—1. Cure, resolution; under proper homœopathic treatment the usual termination.

2. Transition into the chronic form.

3. Ulceration (of the superficial, middle or deeper layers). With the aid of an oblique illumination by means of a biconvex lens, the superficial formation of ulcers, even, may be observed. As long as their bottom remains shiny; the ulcers increase in depth, and photophobia, watering of the eye, and blepharospasm are intense. If the bottom of the ulcer becomes opaque, however (devient legirement opaque); cicatrization begins. The rheumatic ulcera corneæ are more extensive (in periphery), and have uneven edges.

Now and then acute ulcers become chronic. Boyer cured a case, which showed twelve ulcers on the cornea, with *Plumb.* and *Acid nitr.;* hypopyon and iritis existed simultaneously.*

Desmarre's ulcus perforans usually has its seat in the centre of the cornea.

4. The opaque staphyloma is said to be a termination of scrofulous ophthalmia. It is produced when, during perforation of the cornea, the latter softens all over; it is of conical shape. In consequence of it the cornea becomes fibrous, non-transparent, sclerotica-like.

5. Pannus (vasculaire) is developed when the acute symptoms disappear, and it changes the cornea sometimes into a scarlet-colored membrane.

6. Formation of abscesses between the fibrils of the cornea and discharge of pus outwardly or inwardly (*hypopyon*).

7. Iritis, rare, and then always after preceding perforation.

---

We deem it in place to make some remarks at this juncture on Boyer's non-vascular primitive keratitis, especially as the present text-books contain nothing thereupon; at least nothing of a precise character.

---

* He cured a case (within a month), in which five ulcers had already formed upon each cornea, with Silic. and Acid nitr.

The development and course of this inflammation of the cornea without vascular formations is exceedingly slow, lasting months and years, even.

*Symptoms.*—The cornea shows a slight opacity, which soon communicates itself to the whole cornea. The latter, therefore, has an opaque coating, similar to glass that has been breathed upon. Interlamellose thickening of a dirty-white color, which seems to inclose one or more vessels, gradually takes place. At other times we observe real bloody exudations of various extent which are resorbed gradually, *i. e.*, the red-looking exudations become greenish and form a spot often unremovable.

Sometimes the several exudations into the cornea may be demonstrated, while the parts between them remain transparent. These spots are likewise hard to remove.

This form of keratitis is, now and then, entirely confined to the cornea, though the sclerotica always exhibits a bluish tint around the edge of the cornea, yet the remaining portion of the membrane scarcely shows a rosy shine. The conjunctiva palpebrarum remains intact, the mucosa bulbi exhibits but a slight injection in the circumference of the cornea. At a later date the outer membranes and iris become inflamed. Exudations upon the capsula follow, which may be recognized by a comparison with that portion of the cornea remaining transparent. The cornea itself softens, and assumes a form more or less conical. This kind of affection rarely ever ends in ulceration.

It may also happen that the acute phenomena disappear, the exudations become resorbed peripherically, and exhibit in their centre a characteristic appearance.

The patients complain of fog before the eyes, but have no pain; sometimes photophobia and watering of the eye during aggravation.

In certain cases, finally, the retina, also, is irritated, and the process may terminate in real amaurosis.

In most instances digestion is impaired simultaneously; the patients are pale, and have lost flesh. The skin is dry and colorless. At times hardness of hearing is connected with it; oftener a somewhat hoarse voice and swelling of the submaxillary glands.

Prognosis unfavorable on account of the residues mentioned.

Yet, we are able sometimes, at least, to resorb the exudations by homœopathic remedies.

Terminations.—1. Resolution ; rare, slow, and difficult.

2. Spots upon the cornea (usual termination).

3. Staphyloma, very seldom fully developed.

4. Amaurosis.

5. Adhesions of the iris to the capsula are frequent, since the iris often partakes of the inflammation.

The third form of scrofulous ophthalmia, blepharitis ciliaris, we have duly considered above.

The therapia of scrofulous ophthalmia is satisfactory, if we consider that the most torpid cases have been cured by *Calc. carb.;* now and then, by *Calc. jodat.*, *Hep. sulph. c.*, *Acid. nitr.*, and *Arsenicum.* *Mercur.*, *Sulphur.*, *Graphit.* occupy second rank, probably. *Calc. carb.* is most efficacious in dilutions from the 12th to the 30th. *Arsen.* and *Acid. nitr.* cure those cases in which an excessive irritation of the lachrymal ducts exists. *Hepar* is highly praised (applied externally also), by colleague Teller, of Prague, as a specific against remaining spots and opacities of the cornea.* It has also been observed, moreover, that upon the administration of *Apis*, *Senega*, *Baryta*, *Aurum*, and *Bromium*, the cornea rendered non-transparent by exudations (keratitis parenchymatosa) becomes transparent again. *Rhus* and Caustic. would correspond, probably, to the simultaneous rheumatic diathesis, the presence of which proclaims itself by a more intense affection of the fibrous sclerotica. Ulcerous processes come within the sphere of *Silic.* and *Acid. nitr.*

As regards the time, *Bellad.* (6th dil.) would be the most beneficial remedy in the (first) inflammatory period. Later, eight doses of *Calc. carb.*$^{30}$ (one dose daily). If this does not suffice, we shall, probably, be undecided between *Acid. nit.* and *Arsenic*, to return, finally, however, to a preparation of lime, either *Hep. sulph. c.* or *Calc. jod.* or again *Calc. carb.* in a different dose, according to the individuality of the case.

* Internally the 3d trit. of Hep. sulph. calc. (morning and evening) has done, in my hands, extraordinarily good services in subacute cases with simultaneous agglutination of the lids, intense photophobia, and formation of ulcers.

We shall be astonished at the superfluity of all adjuvants, allopathically considered indispensable, such as leeches, purgatives, counter-irritants, eye-lotions, or even the gray mercurial salve, &c. It is precisely in scrofulous ophthalmia that the natura medicatrix, if rationally aided, produces almost miraculous results.

### (*b.*) OPHTHALMIA NEONATORUM.

Since infants, preponderantly scrofulous, are exposed to this disease, for which reason it reaches its highest degree of malignity, we will make the following remarks upon it.

The inflammation appears either as a sporadic, an epidemic, or an endemic affection. Predisposition (to psora), bright light, taking cold, infection of the eyes by impure substances, especially by vaginal secretion—fluor albus—during the passage of the fœtus through the genitals—as well as direct infection from one eye to another, contribute to the full development of the trouble.*

Small crusts around the ciliæ, and a red longitudinal stripe across the upper lid, which is but little swollen, mark out its beginning. Afterwards the swelling becomes more intense. The edge of the lid becomes red, the conjunctiva palpebrarum loosened and velvety (on account of papillar infiltration), and on opening the eyes but a single drop of a wheyish secretion, intermixed with yellowish flakes, is discharged, at first. Later, the upper lid becomes intensely red, often purple, tense, and shiny. The swollen upper lid frequently overlaps the lower entirely (*œdema calidum*).

At this time a secretion resembling bloody water signifies danger.

Finally, the secretion becomes entirely purulent, yellow, even greenish, and often shows traces of blood, produced by the affection of the conjunctiva.

The cornea suffers from a subsequent parenchymatous inflammation, becomes opaque, passes into suppuration, formation of abscesses, perforation, &c., or softens (*malacia*). The lens may drop out, and phthisis bulbi take place, even am-

* Piringers vaccinated with the pus of such children, and obtained positive results.

blyopia on account of the simultaneous irritation of the retina.

THERAPIA.—Homœopathy, we may say without boasting, does not know of any termination of so sad a character. We possess in the RED PRECIPITATE especially, a remedy which answers nearly all demands necessary to enable us to pronounce it a specific.*

Two grains (0, 1) of the 3d trit., morning and evening (or three times daily) suffice even in neglected cases.

This preparation of Mercury corresponds to the most pernicious forms. With *Hep. sulph. calc.*, given in the same manner, and which, probably, still better suits scrofulous individuals, I have obtained results not any less favorable.

Applications of tepid water (small linen compresses) which may be covered with a warm cloth, and remain upon the eyes during the night, advance the cure.

In place of the pure water we may also add to it a few drops of the specific remedy. Thus *Acid. nitri* and *Lycopod.* in low dilutions (3d to 6th) have proved themselves beneficial. A very efficacious remedy is ten drops of the first dilution of *Acid. nitri* with two grammes of *Spirit. vin. rectif.* Of this solution fifteen drops in a saucerful of water to moisten compresses with. *Sulph.*, *Calc. carb.*, and other remedies are likewise not to be despised. Yet, I have successfully treated the most intense forms of that fearful ophthalmia by the remedies first mentioned. Indeed, these cases were frequently such as had been maltreated or neglected in the most inexcusable manner, and in which perforation of and ulceration upon the highly inflamed cornea gave occasion to fears of the worst kind.

It is self-evident that we will treat a slight inflammation of the eye by *Acon.* or *Bellad.* (and a few doses of *Calc. carb.* or *Lycopod.* at longer intervals), without taking refuge forthwith with the precipitate, &c. The further course of the inflammation alone indicates the subsequent selection of that remedy.

* We mention here that, according to Adam Fischer, the white precipitate of mercury (in the form of the Ung. hydr. pracc. albi) is said to be specific also in common, scrofulous ophthalmia (with the "scrofulo-vascular ribbon" called after A. Fischer).

The advice of allopathic ophthalmologists, to wash out the eyes with lukewarm water repeatedly (from three to four hours), and with cold water in case of intense production of heat, deserves some notice; but, on the other hand, we are inclined to consider the solutions of Nitrate of Silver (as strong as 15 grains to ℥j) as well as those of Sulphate of Copper, as causes of the many fatal terminations.

NOTE.—The chronic, croupous blennorrhœa of the conjunctiva described by Payr in his classical treatise on the diseases of the conjunctiva (A. H. Z., 78, 71), which appears in form of an affection of the texture of the corpus papillare, in consequence of which the conjunctiva assumes a granulated (frog-spawn-like) appearance, according to the experiences of the same physician, finds its remedy likewise in *Hydr. præcip. rubr.*, a fact that may allow us, probably, to infer a certain relation between the two diseases.

### 2. *Scrofulous Inflammation of the Ear—Otitis Scrofulosa.*

Here we must distinguish two forms:

(*a.*) The catarrhal inflammation of the meatus auditorius externus—*otitis catarrh. externa.*

(*b.*) The muco-membranous inflammation of the middle ear; *inflammatio cat. s. catarrhus auris mediæ, otitis catarrh. interna.*

#### (*a.*) THE INFLAMMATION OF THE EXTERNAL EAR.

*Otitis Catarrhalis Externa.*

Catarrhal inflammation of the external ear-passage commences with a slight itching, afterwards burning pain in the meatus, the pain being ameliorated momentarily by inserting the finger. While the pain diminishes, a discharge of a serous, afterwards creamy, flocculent character, yellowish in color and of sweetish or ammoniac smell, shows itself. Thus we observe a process somewhat similar to that of common coryza, or of a gonorrhœic inflammation even. The secretion hardens at the external ear to yellowish crusts, decreases or increases periodically, and becomes more profuse during the night. If the discharge stops, the secretion of ear-wax, thus far absent, reappears. A slight disturbance of hearing is always present, and roaring in the ears usually. The membrana tympani, in the neighborhood of the handle of the malleus, is reddened. The inflamed, serous, infiltrated lining of the meatus is loosened in its tissue, covered here and there with small papulæ, vesicles or pustules, has a flaky, villous appearance, and finally swells up to such a degree as to make the opposite walls touch each other; a state of things which sometimes renders the inspection of the membrana tympani utterly impossible.

Since the membrana tympani remains unaffected, the prognosis of this catarrhal, aural affection is favorable. I should compare it to herpes conjunctivæ or scrofulo-pustular ophthalmia. If this analogy is tenable, the remedies against both affections will be the same. And, in fact, *Calc. carb.* (besides *Lycopod.*, *Mercur.*, *Sulph.*, *Hepar sulph. calc.*) is in place here as well as there.

Scrofulous otitis inclines toward a chronic course, and changes, now and then, into genuine blennorrhœa, mostly with an acrid, offensive secretion. The membrana tympani is apt to lose its lustre and to thicken. Upon longer duration papulous excrescences may form, now starting at the walls of the meatus, now at the membrana tympani. The disease seldom affects originally both ears simultaneously, yet, at a later date, transplants itself almost always from one ear to the other, or, perhaps, alternates between the two.

Hence, the scrofulous external catarrhs of the ear exhibit the characteristic that they do not very easily terminate spontaneously, but drag out in the form of a so-called otorrhœa. According to Rau, in catarrhal otitis, not only perforation of the membr. tymp. never takes place, but also no secondary inflammation of the periosteum of the meatus, of the mastoid process, or of the brain, even such as are admitted by many to occur. We may infer the scrofulous character of such cases of otitis, especially when they set in after exanthemata (scarlatina; measles).

It is a pleasing sign that more recent therapeutics (Rau, Politzer) warns against the intense cauterizations. It is true it deems injections of metallic salts (Cupr. acet., Zinc. acet., Plumb. acet. and sulph., Argent. nitric.) to be remedies, yet

Politzer himself admits that by means of too strong injections one obtains a result exactly contrary to that he aims at, a more profuse discharge.* The injections ought not to occasion any burning.

Rau deems medicated injections and the dropping of Infus. chamom., millefolii, Liquamen myrrhæ, into the ears, the painting of the inner ear with Bals. peruv., the fumigations of Mastix, Olibanum, &c., absolutely harmful.

It is most remarkable, however, that Rau (especially in case of a simultaneous and offensive discharge) recommends lime-water, the carbonate of lime being with us the remedy most frequently applied.

### (*b*.) THE INFLAMMATION OF THE INNER EAR.

*Otitis Catarrhalis Interna.*

How much this inflammation interests us here is plain from the words of the author mentioned above, who says: "On more careful examination we shall usually observe that the cause of the muco-membranous inflammation of the middle ear is intimately connected with a scrofulous disposition. There are families in which hardly one member remains free from this disease of the middle ear. Children of this predisposition are exposed to eruptions on the head and face, but especially to frequent slight attacks of angina and coryza, under the influence of which the disease develops now and then entirely imperceptibly; or an acute exanthematic eruption, hooping-cough, catarrhal fever, causes a sudden appearance of otit. interna." Rau, as a rule, regards otit. int. to be one of the most frequent disturbances of the ear existing.† Besides the cavum tympani, the tuba Eustachii, and the processus mastoideus participate in the affection. The catarrh, in fact, is wont to start at the tuba Eustach.‡ Hardness of hearing, which may approach to complete deafness, more in-

* This was the case of a pale, feeble child, for whom a representative of the school of "exact medicine" prescribed 3.0 (say three grammes) of Zinc. sulph. (to 100 gramm. of water) as an injection.

† Of 1000 patients, afflicted with aural diseases, he saw 352 who suffered from inflammation of the mucosa of the middle ear.

‡ v. Tscharner, of 200 patients afflicted with aural diseases, found 62 who suffered from inflammation of the tub. Eustach.

tense in the morning, and dependent upon changes of weather, is never absent. Fresh catarrhal affections (a slight coryza, the most insignificant beginning of an angina) forthwith occasion an aggravation. The air-douche, which, in acute forms, causes an unpleasant sensation, but improves the hearing almost immediately as soon as the air enters the cavum tympani, alone gives positive information.

The acute form, almost always connected with other catarrhal affections, coryza, cough, hoarseness, &c., mostly begins with hardness of hearing, roaring in the ears, sensation of fulness, and heaviness in the ear, dulness in the head, and especially with stitches running from the neck to the ear. In case of a milder attack these symptoms imperceptibly disappear after a few days with an increased mucous discharge from the nose and pharynx, the air entering sometimes suddenly into the reopened cavum tympani with a loud report. If the mucus collected in the cavum tympani cannot be evacuated on account of the swelling of the tuba Eustachii, the hardness of hearing remains not only unimproved, but increases. Perforation of the membrana tympani, destruction of the ossicula auditus, caries of the proc. mastoid, do not belong to this form, and their enumeration here is owing to a confounding of the trouble with periostitis cavi tympani.

### (*c*.) PERIOSTITIS AURIS MEDIÆ.

This affection must also be mentioned here, since as otit. int. it manifests a characteristic pathological picture, and there cannot be any doubt as to its independence. Rau calls it "the most important aural disease," endangering not only the organ affected, but also life itself. Usually departing from the membrana tympani, and simultaneously attacking all parts of the middle ear, this inflammation affects, above all, the periosteum. Without remaining confined to the middle ear, it passes almost invariably over to the tuba Eustach., and the cells of the mastoid process, is frequently communicated to the labyrinth, and may transplant itself to the meninges and even to the brain.

With the commencement of the purulent, exceedingly offensive discharge we always find the membrana tympani perforated, sometimes destroyed to a great extent. In the acute and chronic form the discharge, coloring the silver probe with a blackish hue, is mixed with granules of bone, and at a later date, the corpuscula auditus may be expelled. This, however, does not always occur. But if the caries makes any progress, a soft, fluctuating swelling, with the color of the integuments unchanged, appears upón the proc. mastoid, almost without exception, which, settling in a downward direction, frequently opens at a lower place, whereupon the destruction of the bony parts may be ascertained by the probe. At the appearance of the purulent discharge from the meatus, the cerebral symptoms (vertigo, one-sided pain in the head, weakness of memory, sleepiness) often disappear temporarily, and the hearing often improves to a considerable degree. Notwithstanding, however, the patient is in constant danger, since fresh inflammatory attacks frequently take place without any cause known, which at times occasion death by apoplexy very unexpectedly.

The disease mostly appearing before puberty, is usually connected with a scrofulous diathesis; so that the latter has to be considered the predisposing momentum. In many cases chronic exanthemata with reflex action upon the meat. audit. ext. in form of otit. catarrh. ext., appear previously; after the disappearance of which the disease often breaks out suddenly.

(*d.*)

Of less importance is the periostitis of the meat. aud. ext., for the diagnosis of which the silver probe suffices.

(*e.*)

The inflammation of the membrana tympani also occurs preponderantly with the scrofulous, especially as a secondary pathological process, resulting from the inflammation of the external meatus and the middle portion of the ear. A purulent discharge, connected with hardness of hearing, frequently is the first symptom arousing the attention of the patient. Pain, if existing, is but transient in case of decrease or discontinuation of the discharge. The secretion of ear-wax is regularly suppressed. The membrana tympani always thickens in course of time. Partial destructions happen. Granulations of polypous form; rarely genuine polypi.

Now, as regards the therapeutics of all these conditions, the homœopathic method of healing has the great advantage of never contributing anything to the forcible suppression of the otorrhœa, always to be considered as a beneficial crisis, though of an incomplete character. If physicians, such as Hufeland, warn against the suppression of cutaneous scrofulous eruptions, how much more ought this advice to apply with regard to the internal, catarrhal, and periosteal otorrhœæ, connected, as they are, with the brain in a manner more or less demonstrable. Authorities in otiatrics admit at the same time that, after the cessation of an otorrhœa, pain, hardness of hearing and affections of the brain may appear, and when notwithstanding they cling to the Lapis infern. divinus, Cupr. sulph., Plumb. acet., &c., they occupy the position of those Athenians of whom it was said that "they knew well enough what was right, but did not do it."

As homœopath, moreover, one needs not be a specialist and yet may make excellent cures of (scrofulous) diseases of the ear. In order to apply the right remedy, it is fully sufficient to know, whether a catarrh or a carious process is present, and whether it bears the acute or chronic character. The quality of the secretion is easily ascertained, as well as the seat of the affection. From the above remarks it is plain that the five usual forms: catarrhal inflammation of the external meatus, cavum tympani, periosteal inflammation of the meat. extern. and cavum tympani and, finally, meningitis must be distinguished, and how.

Our suppuration-remedies, if I am permitted to use the expression, act just as surely upon that portion before as upon that behind the membr. tympani.

It has already been mentioned that in the treatment of mechanical conditions (narrowing of the tuba Eustach.), we cannot do without certain mechanical aids, such as catheterization, air-douche, &c.

Besides, it has also been said that every disturbance of the ear finds its analogon in a corresponding affection of the eye; hence, the specific therapia, if fixed with regard to one organ, would likewise apply to the analogous condition of the other.

In the treatment of scrofulous persons suffering from diseases of the ear, it is important to know that even the homœopathic cure often requires a long time, weeks and months, but that nevertheless the prognosis is not unfavorable. We could mention more than one pernicious case in which under allopathic treatment polypous growths, profuse, putrid discharge, general decline and a considerable degree of hardness of hearing had made their appearance, where notwithstanding, *Calcar.*, *Silic.*, and *Mercur.* (the first and third in their different preparations) were fully sufficient to master the pathological processes, *Ferrum jod.* sach. has to be given, occasionally, as an intercurrent remedy, and as a drug improving the constitution.

Iodine vapors have been lauded in chronic inflammation of the membr. tymp. developing upon a scrofulous bottom. (Tinct. Iodii, gtt. 2–6 to from 3 to 4 ounces of water) (Tscharner, Schw. Zeitschr., 1851.)

### 3. *Scrofulous Affections of the Mucosa of the Nose.*

The scrofulous affections of the nose, like those of the ear, have also to be distinguished as acute and chronic.

#### (*a.*) CORYZA

Is too well known to be described here. I will mention, however, that the cure of the chronic form is often of great importance, scrofula in its totality not rarely being removed with it. (Kafka.)

Besides the usual remedies (*Sulph.*, *Hep. sulph. calc.*) *Graphit.* and *Arget. nitric.* have effected results when profuse, puri-sanguineous nasal secretion existed, the sense of smell was blunted, and the nasal mucosa appeared sore and ulcerated. (Eczemata at the nasal openings and upper lip.)

In case of a bloated face, swollen nose and upper lip, offensive discharge, dried-up crusts in the interior of the nose, ulcerated nasal openings, *Calc. carb.* 6. If this be without result, *Silic.* or *Mercur. præcip. rub.* 3. *Aurum mur. natr.* and *Kali. bichrom.*, and lastly, *Arsenicum* (*Lachesis*). *Arsenicum:* anæmia of a high grade, œdematous swellings of the lower extremities, emaciation, increased thirst, eczemata, swelling of the submaxillary and axillary glands.

Among the most important scrofulous affections of the nose we count:

### (*b.*) OZÆNA.

Formation of ulcers and fetid smell accompany it. If but the latter is present, the trouble is Oz. *spuria*, Oz. *non-ulcerosa*, only.

Complete or but partial loss of smell, now a light-colored, fluid, or reddish, now a yellow and thick quality of the secretion intermixed with streaks of blood, frequently drying up to *crusts*, and the *insufferable smell* of the discharge characterize the ulcerous ozæna.

Sometimes we can observe the ulcers directly; any portion of the nasal mucosa may become affected.

The obstinacy of the disease, frequently defying all therapeutics, is owing to the participating of cartilages and bones in the pathological process.

Though *Calc. carb.*, *Hep. sulph.*, *Phosph.*, *Graph.*, *Pulsat.*, *Nux vom.*, *Silic.*, and *Sulphur* have been recommended, they nevertheless not rarely fail.*

We may explain the recommendation of the various remedies in this way that (by means of a remedy, or without it, even) the subsequent amelioration was taken for a cure too readily. We have seen such improvements after *Graph.*, *Arsenic.*, &c., but no radical cures. The same holds good of *Kal. hydroj.*, which, in doses of one grain daily, still deserves most confidence. Nasal suctions of Chlorine-water even do not dispel the penetrant "mouldy or caseo-putrid smell."

Kafka has recorded (Hom. Therap., ii, 743, case of ozæna of eight years' standing) a cure by *Hydr. præcip. rubr.* 3 internally (externally the crusts that could be reached were besmeared with *Unguent. hydr. præcip. rubr.* (0.06 : 2.0) ). The difficulty of a cure is owing, no doubt, to the peculiar construction of the nose, and (besides the partaking of cartilage and bone in the pathological process) to the arrest of the ulcerous secretion dependent thereupon.

Dr. Baer cured a girl, æt. 13, with *Aur. met.*, who had already suffered for a long time to the greatest torment of her

* Thus Dr. Gentzke also describes (A. H. Z., 22, 9) an interesting case of Oz. scrof. in a female servant, æt. 22, and frankly confesses that Puls , Merc., Phosph., Aur., Thuj., Sulph., and Calc. carb., had not improved it any. He closes with a modest quid hic faciendum ?

friends from a horribly smelling, nasal discharge of a viscid, purulent character, and very offensive breath. Her appearance was almost ruddy, yet somewhat "scrofulous" (A. H. Z., 54, 1).

We repeat that ozæna is apt to show a very malignant character, but that the want of therapeutic success is owing to homœopaths, rather than homœopathy. It is an interesting fact, however, that the remedy deserving of most confidence, the *red precipitate*, is specific also against ophthalmia neonatorum, a disease which may be marked out as an expression of a scrofulous constitution not any less obstinate. We may be inclined to infer that both diseases belong, perhaps, to scrofulous affections, modified by syphilitic antecedents.

### (*c*.) POLYPI OF THE MUCOUS MEMBRANE.

A peculiar termination of the chronic muco-membranous inflammation is the polypous growth. They are distinguished according to their consistency as fibrinous and mucous polypi. Besides the aural mucosa, the nasal, especially, produces polypi, which recur most obstinately in spite of surgical extirpation, or their removal by torsion. The appearance of polypi is mostly identical with intense scrofulosis, and especially with that form of it modified by more advanced age. The soft polypi start at the subcutaneous tissue or perichondrium.

In case of larger polypi we observe loss of smell, gaping of the mouth, nasal voice, frequent but ineffective blowing of the nose. Firm, fleshy polypi, may displace the lachrymal canal, and thus occasion watering of the eyes; or since they affect the tuba Eustach., hardness of hearing. Mucous, purulent coryza, and ulceration even, may accompany the presence of polypi.

If the polypus is seated high up, the diagnosis is facilitated by closing up one nasal opening, and requesting the patient to blow through the other. We recognize the presence of polypi by the impossibility of air passing through it.

THERAPIA.—Whoever denies the efficacy of homœopathic remedies, sees himself confined, as already said, to incomplete surgical aid. Yet we possess drugs capable of counteracting the polypous process, among which belong, especially, CALC. CARB. and TEUCRIUM MARUM. Aside from these, according to the individuality of the case, *Conium*, *Phosph.*, *Aurum*, *Bellad.*, *Graphit.*, *Mercur.*, *Acid nitri*, *Silic.*, *Sulph.*, *Staphisagria.* (Journal de la Médec. Hom., 1, 5). Polypi frequently appear contemporaneously with those ominous chronic swellings of the tonsils, which, likewise, have to be considered as an undeniable, partial phenomenon of general scrofulosis. *Calc. jod.* has proved itself efficacious against these tonsilar swellings. We request homœopaths to try it against polypi.

### 4. *Mucosa of the Mouth.*

The connection between the affections to be mentioned here and scrofulosis is more difficult to prove than that with regard to the eye, ear, and nose. Yet such affections do exist, notwithstanding. Among them we count:

#### (*a.*) THE CATARRHAL INFLAMMATION OF THE MUCOSA.

*Stomatitis Catarrhalis.*

It is connected with redness and increased secretion. The tongue looks as if it were covered with a thick layer of raspberry syrup. On longer duration a white coat appears upon it. The children do not like to have any portion of the mouth touched. Mucus always flows down the corners of the mouth, excoriating them, reddening the chin, and soiling the clothes. The mucus is wont to react acidly.

When redness and soreness have lasted a few days, small vesicles, as real exudations, in appearance and course much resembling herpes (labialis), rise up at the mucosa of the tongue, gums, lips, and cheeks. They soon burst and leave small, superficial ulcers with a yellowish-white bottom, increase in the first few days in all directions, become confluent, and produce ulcerated surfaces of some extent, especially at the edge of the tongue, and the mucosa of the lower lip.

*These ulcers never have a peculiar smell.*

THERAPIA.—*Acid. nitr.* when small ulcers are present. *Mercur.* in case of great flow of saliva. But from the internal and external application of *Borax*, also (1st or 2d trit.), beneficial results have been obtained.

A characteristic fetid smell we find in

### (*b.*) STOMACACE,

which is not accompanied by increased secretion of the buccal mucosa, as stomatitis catarrh. is, from which, according to some authors, it may develop, and which occasions ulcerative processes of greater extent. It shows but little inclination to heal spontaneously; swelling, ulcers, and smell, without treatment, may last for months; the teeth become loose and fall out, and the children become emaciated to a dangerous degree.

I should compare Stom. *catarrh*, to coryza with its termination into ozæna *benigna* (*non-ulcerans*), stomacace to ozæna *maligna*.

The subsequent course (after the forerunners of simple stomatitis) of stomacace is that the parts adjoining the gums, are infected by contact, and suffer the same changes. The mucosa of the cheeks swells considerably, so much so as to show the impression of the several teeth upon it. The same is true of the tongue (swelling of the cervical glands).

Alfred Vogel says: "*Calomel*, in children, produces a disease of the mouth that cannot be distinguished in any way from stomacace, unless the absence of contagiousness of stomac. mercurialis, above mentioned, is to be set up as a diagnostic sign."

By this remark, and the fact that *Mercur.* is homœopathically indispensable in stomacace, we again see the correctness of the law of the simile confirmed.

Besides *Acid. nitri.*, *Sulph.*, and against stomac. catarrh., *Borax* is indicated. Since Borax is used allopathically, even, against catarrhal inflammation of the buccal mucosa; there could, as regards stomacace, also be no objection raised homœopathically against *Kali chloric.;* especially, as according to the testimony of able allopathic therapeutists, it is said to be the most specific remedy for it, existing.

### (*c.*) APHTHÆ.

A form of stomatitis connected with the formation of fungi (oidium albicans) which depends upon predominant acidity.

Aphthæ are related to scrofulosis, probably, as tinea favosa is, of which Jousset says:

"Quant à la teigne faveuse, décrite si longtemps comme une affection scrofuleuse, elle est rangée aujourd'hui parmi les affections parasitaires, seulement les scrofuleux offrent un terrain très favorable à son développement."

THERAPIA.—As against stomat. catarrh. good results have been obtained by *Borax* (1st and 2d trit.). Everything containing sugar (even milk, on account of its containing sugar and caseine) is to be avoided, since aphthæ owe their origin to a surplus of acidity.*

## II. ORGANS OF RESPIRATION.

### 1. *Croup*,

Though not a genuine form of scrofula, preponderantly affects scrofulous children. Kafka has observed that the torpid course of croup, especially, is owing to a scrofulous constitution. For quite different reasons we should claim croup to be a disease almost specifically scrofulous; we mean on account of the efficacy of the remedies, successfully employed against it, all of which are antiscrofulosa of first rank.

(Torpid) Croup is cured by the ametals or metalloids of anorganic constitution. Except those existing in gas-form (oxygen, hydrogen, nitrogen) almost every one of them has been successfully used against this malignant and pernicious disease of children. *Sulphur* (as *Hep. sulph. calc.*), *Phosph.*, *Carbon*, *Spongia*, *Iodium* among the solid metalloids, and lastly, the fluid *Brom.* which plays a role exceedingly important.†

The distinction between *spurious* and *genuine* croup is of subordinate value, for the latter may develop from the former.

---

* Some refer scrofulosis, as is well known, to a surplus of acidity, and thus explain the usefulness of alkalies.

† Dr. Sybel of Aschersleben observed cases of angina membran., in which Acon., Hep., Spong., Iod., Brom., Ant. tart., could not prevent the fatal termination. Upon theoretical grounds, *i. e.*, supported by the pathogenesis of the remedy, he proposes Ammon. caustic. internally, and to be inhaled by the nose.

In the fatal cases, referred to above, the cough was absent almost entirely.

Hence, every inflammation of the larynx, accompanied by the characteristic croupy sound, is to be treated as croup from the very beginning. The prognosis is unfavorable in the highest degree, and the formation of real membranous exudations is to be expected most surely, if tonsilar diphtheritis precedes the croupous process. But, then, we may be assured that the characteristic chronic swelling of the tonsils, so often observed with the scrofulous, has already existed previously. The action of the skin or nasal mucosa, present or absent, is also of prognostic importance, since the appearance of sweat and coryza (especially if the latter had stopped suddenly) point to a crisis, and dispel all fear of a plastic exudation. Finally, from the continuing hoarseness and aphonia we may almost always infer that the croup is genuine (membranous), just as a case of scarlatina, diagnostically doubtful, documents itself, *a posteriori*, by the desquamation and peeling off of the epidermis.

Although we always prefer the record of cases treated to pathological remarks of a lengthy and general character, and shall present in the course of our treatise more than one such cure of croup; we will yet give in the following a few additional items as regards its pathology.

Sometimes, but proportionally rarely, croup begins suddenly with a rough, barking cough and difficulty of breathing.

It is mostly preceded by forerunners, such as hoarseness, sharp cough, catarrh of the larynx and pharynx. Signs of a diphtheritic affection of the latter. Weakness, ill humor, fever, loss of appetite, difficulty of breathing during sleep.

The increase of the trouble manifests itself by the roughness of the paroxysmal cough, the pain in the larynx, extinction of voice, or by a violent, almost always nocturnal attack of suffocation with a whistling, short, and tormenting cough.

If at this period amelioration does not set in, the difficulty of breathing increases amid the most powerful efforts, reddening and paling and swelling of the face, and paroxysms which are interrupted by intense exhaustion, though of but momentary duration. A few hours later, general collapse; a pulse growing smaller and smaller, secondary emphysema of the lungs, and death set in as early as on the first day.

But in most cases the first attack remains moderate yet,

although the cough is rough and suppressed, the voice weak, hoarse and interrupted by whistling sounds; the patient falls asleep again, but breathes with whistling noises, and shows restlessness during sleep with repeated starting. On the next day there is a decided amelioration of the phenomena, but still greater weakness remains. In the course of the same day, or the night following, or on the next day, even, paroxysms of suffocation again set in which become more and more violent.

In the intervals between the attacks we may observe mostly pain in the region of the larynx, heaving and whistling respiration, now restlessness, now a semi-soporous condition together with a very accelerated pulse and increased temperature. At a later period the paroxysms come at shorter intervals, continue longer, and are interrupted only by soporous exhaustion; the lung begins to distend itself emphysematically, and continuous dyspnœa with a cyanotic appearance shows itself during the intervals, even. Though the attacks themselves gradually grow more moderate now, yet the respiratory impediment becomes more and more permanent, and slight jerks and more violent convulsions appear in addition. In some cases pseudo-membranes are coughed up, always with relief, which, however, usually is but temporary. Now and then, a mucous and viscid liquid is evacuated by vomiting with some benefit.

In some cases, not so exceedingly rare, the symptoms decrease, it is true; the breathing becomes more free, and more rest is obtained, yet the pulse remains extraordinarily frequent, and though the respiratory impediment is removed, the sopor increases, and death occurs from gradual collapse with or without the addition of œdema pulmonum.

Therapia.—There cannot be the slightest doubt but that the prognosis of croup is not as hopeless under homœopathic as under allopathic treatment. Indeed, we need but take up allopathic textbooks of a recent date and more enlightened, to perceive that the aids, formerly considered indispensable, such as venesection, counter-irritants, cauterizations, and others, are condemned; at the same time, however, so great a helplessness becomes apparent that things of the most contradictory nature are recommended. There a Wunderlich, even, does not scorn the idea of appealing "without hesitation," now to mercurial salve, now to inhalations of chloroform, now to moschus, now to opium "in large doses," now to asafœtid., now to tracheotomy. Indeed, in order to make the irony complete, he mentions Hep. sulph., even, in doses from one to six grains. In the latter recommendation we see the obtuse presentiment of the possibility of a better therapia of croup than the present one. Yet, there is no mention made of remedies, such as Spong., Iod., Brom., Phosph., and Kali bichrom., so important in the most severe cases of genuine croup.

Nowhere is the recommendation of medicines connected with so great a responsibility as in croup. For the most tortuous death would be the consequence of an erroneous treatment. Our recommendation of the homœopathic therapia, aside from its being based upon numerous and trustworthy reports of others, rests, therefore, upon clinical observations of our own. At this juncture we will not fail to remark, 1, that we entirely agree with Dr. Weil's views, that when one declares that he has treated croup in one and the same individual, five or more times, the disease was not membranous croup, but pseudo-croup; 2, that the homœopathic specifica, though efficacious, are not able to arrest a case of croup at once, but sometimes let us wait very long, indeed, for the final removal of the ominous attacks.

Moreover, in case of a malignant course of the disease, we would not like to do without the wet bandage around the throat as an auxiliary means. It is remarkable how well it is borne at the height of the disease. Upon the whole, we have in the natural curative instinct a guide for the various curative apparatuses. The cold bandage, if not appropriate any longer, is refused. The same holds good of inhalations, which, likewise, at a certain period and stage, prove themselves very beneficial (S. LXIII). Thus I let *Iodium* (1 drop to circa four grammes of water) or *Bromium*, or *Hep. sulph. calc.*, even, vapor off, or be inhaled with benefit as long as no resistance is made.

The wet bandage is apt to produce sweat, which, starting at the throat, spreads over the rest of the body. But it is the sweat, especially, which is absent in membranous croup; the skin remains hot and dry. When warm sweat is present, cold water ought not to be applied.

Spurious croup, which, fortunately, is observed much oftener, is cured by *Aconit.* (within the first twenty-four hours), and *Hep. sulph. calc.* (Kafka), or *Spongia.* If the crisis (loose cough, sweat, discharge from the nose) has set in after Aconitum, *Bellad.* is well indicated for the second day. Hot, sweetened milk, drank in large quantities within the first hours of a sudden attack of croup (usually at night) assists the crisis. It is difficult to give TENABLE indications as regards the several croup-remedies. If we look at the respective reports of cures, we find that, in most desperate cases, the metalloids named, *Iod.*, *Brom.*, *Spong.*, have almost always been given (and in this fact we notice, in contradistinction to the allopathic school, the observance of a uniform principle); but, at other times, it required *Kal. bichrom.*, *Tr. Sambuci*, *Kaolin*, *Tart. stib.* (in hom. trit.), or *Phosph.* (applied locally, even), before the disease was broken. It is a disadvantage that in this disease we feel less inclined than almost in any other, to allow the remedy to develop its full action, since otherwise the danger might reach an incontrollable height.

Hoarseness, amounting to aphonia, pathognomonic of genuine croup, as we may say, sometimes requires an especial after-treatment, lest it may continue for months even. *Lycopod.*, *Caustic.*, *Graph.*, *Phosph.*, *Silic.* would be the remedies to be tried. Also, hot milk and Seltzer water as auxiliary means.

### 2. *The Bronchial Catarrh of the Scrofulous*

Characterizes itself by its chronic course—its appearance during childhood, the partaking of the lungs in the affection—an occurrence that may easily happen—and the great quantity of sputa of a sero-purulent quality. On account of the relation of scrofulosis to tuberculosis such catarrhs ought to be watched with the greatest care. The children have mostly fever with it, lose flesh, and auscultation often shows surprising differences in the resonance between the right and left pulmonary apex. A peculiar shortness of breathing, always suspicious, and signs of disturbed digestion, mental depression, and changed disposition, are always present.

THERAPIA.—*Sulphur*, especially, is able to prevent the evil terminations of this catarrh, and to resolve the infiltrations in the pulmonary tissue. Afterwards *Phosph.*,* *Mercur.*, *Hep. sulph. calc.*, *Calc. carb.*, *Silic.*, *Lycopod.*, but also *Pulsat.*, *Scill.*, and *China*, &c., effect much.

*Ipecac.* is likewise most valuable, especially in case of simultaneous chronic looseness of the bowels, and a spasmodic character of the cough, but mostly is efficacious only in form of a weak infusion.

Finally, we must not forget *Kal. carb.*, which plays so important a part in incipient phthisis, and is indicated in case of predominant stitching pains in the breast; hence, in case of pleuritic symptoms, shortness of breathing, especially in childhood, and with females. Hemorrhages would point to *Kal. carb.* all the more. I use the 3d trituration (morning and evening 0.1 gramme) with very great benefit against the respective chronic or subacute pulmonary catarrh of scrofulous persons, in whom I suspect a predisposition to tuberculosis. The characteristic swelling of the tonsils and crusty soreness of the nasal mucosa (in the region of the nasal openings) mostly existed simultaneously with those catarrhs.

In such cases too much importance cannot be placed upon a corresponding change of air, a residence in a country, sunny and rich in pine forests, and upon the milk-cure, &c. (milk of asses and goats, &c., warm as it is drawn from the bag).

## III. ORGANS OF DIGESTION.

"Chronic catarrhs of the stomach and intestines, with paresis of the intestinal musculature," according to Wunderlich, are troubles not rarely found with the scrofulous. These conditions are either of a more transient nature (in which now constipation, now diarrhœa, has to be met) or continuous,

* I found Phosph. repeatedly specific when breathing was so impeded that one felt as if he should help the children in their respiratory efforts; hence, when a certain degree of dyspnœa existed. Also Lycopod., in case of so-called consonant râles, when a concomitant noise, like the sound from an organ, or a whistling was heard while breathing. So in the cough accompanying influenza. Scilla (in a low dilution, a few drops at a time) in case of excessive mucous rattling, when the children cannot get control over the mucus. Here China (in a low dilution, or the mother-tincture even) is also indicated.

and then of evil omen. An affection of the mesenterial glands, and, in consequence, degeneration of those organs takes place, and such children die miserably under the symptoms of a follicular enteritis or chronic atrophia, probably in combination with ascites. The nosological picture of such an abdominal localization of scrofula we find most instructively given in the curative results of Baryta mur. and Arsenic (see those). There we regularly find also scrofulous concomitants, such as swollen glands of the neck, cutaneous eruptions of the head, &c. The character and course of abdominal scrofula is drawn nearly as precisely as is that of scrofulous ophthalmia or ozæna.

Therapia.—Aside from the remedies mentioned, *Calc. carb.* and *Phosph.*, and in those cases characterized by eruptions of all kinds, especially furunculous abscesses on the head and trunk, *Sulph.* and *Silicea* will suffice, perhaps. *Carb. veg.*, also, may come under consideration in atrophia infantum, especially if decided symptoms of scrofulosis were present previously (see cures by Carbo veg.).

Note.—Probably hydrocephalus acutus may, with more propriety than any other disease, be compared to this manifestation of scrofulosis; and it seems that, at a certain period of time, the nature of the child remains, so to say, undecided before this alternation, until an external incidental cause (a mistake in diet, chilling of the head, &c.) influences it to decide itself for this or that cavity (abdominal or cranial).

---

## *C.*—The Glandular System.

### 1. *The Lymphatic Glands.*

That the lymphatic glands frequently are affected by scrofula, and become the seat of abscesses, is not to be wondered at in view of the predominant significance of this anatomical system with regard to scrofulosis in general; for swellings of the neighboring glands never fail to appear in case of any extensive peripheric localization of that diathesis.

We may distinguish between inflammatory, scrofulous, and non-inflammatory infiltrations.

We observe the inflammations most frequently behind the ears, at the lower jaw, neck, in the axilla, more rarely at the inguinal region. According to the degree of the inflammation, its extension over the subcutaneous connective tissue, and the number of the glands affected, such inflammations are accompanied, more or less, by febrile symptoms, local pains, and nightly exacerbation. They mostly terminate in suppuration, sometimes after the previous appearance of severe chills. Not unfrequently a complete cure follows upon the spontaneous or artificial evacuation of pus; the inflammations often recur at short intervals, or appear slowly with but slight inflammatory symptoms; then the inflammatory infiltrations remain at an incomplete stage of development, and, by mostly spreading from one portion of the gland to another, and thus forming a connected chain of suppurative foci, pass over into the process of softening not before weeks or months, occasioning an unhealthy look, loss of flesh and strength, and leaving behind disfiguring and contracted cicatrices. In other cases a suppuration-focus develops only at a circumscribed spot of the glands, infiltrated by inflammation; the pus, however, does not perforate the glandular capsula, but thickens and passes over into caseous metamorphosis. In consequence of these hard knots the glands may assume an irregular, tuberous appearance. If the cheesy content of the gland calcifies it acts like a foreign body.

The non-inflammatory infiltration of the lymphatic glands consists in chronic swelling of the separate glands, which occasion neither pain nor redness, mostly feel like round, oblong, smooth or hard bodies, and often attain to a considerable size. If several glands standing in a row, or forming clusters, become scrofulously infiltrated simultaneously, or in succession, they frequently appear as knotty ropes, or as disfiguring not smooth but tuberous packages. Resorption can take place only, when the glandular contents (infiltration) are *cellular* (increase of cells—Virchow), but hardly ever in case they be lardaceous or chalky. Therefore, we cannot always expect, as we have said above, cheesy or albuminous contents. Yet, the idea of scrofula does not agree with that of cellular infiltration.

With many practitioners, however, the appearance of glandular infiltrations is taken to be a pathognomonic symptom of scrofula.

THERAPIA.—The acute, scrofulous glandular inflammations are treated with *Bellad.*, *Aconit.*, *Mercur.*, or other remedies corresponding to the individual case. If abscesses threaten to form, *Hep. sulph. calc.*, *Mercur.*, *Silic.* If the opening does not close up, but continually discharges a watery fluid, *Caustic.* (pledgets of lint saturated with it) is well suited. After *Sil.*, *Phosph.* will often be indicated, to which Kafka rightly attributes a vitalizing effect upon the paralyzed curative activity. The same author recommends *Kal. hydrojod.* 2d or 3d, externally and internally, or *Conium*, twice or three times daily, in case of want of reaction in the purple, swollen, and nearly painless glands, which do not pass on either into suppuration or resorption.

*Silic.* and *Acid. nitri.* modify too profuse suppuration. They correspond also (besides *Phosph.*) to torpid (weak in reaction) scrofulous ulcers, such as may develop from abscesses in the lymphatic glands.

In case of an ichorous, offensive discharge, *Arsenic.*, *Kreosot.*, Asafœt. However, the most sovereign remedy against indolent non-inflammatory glands is Iodium and Kal. hydrojod. *Sep.*, *Con.*, *Baryt. carb.*, without excluding *Phosph.* and *Silic.*, may be applied, if simultaneous coughing up of blood exists, or if frail individuals pass, at the same time, through the period of evolution. *Carb. an.*, finally, is a remedy not to be despised in benignant as well as malignant glandular affections of the most various kind.

If the remedies mentioned are of no avail, we may infer a lardaceous or colloid content of the glands. Then *Brom.* and *Aurum mur.*, in spite of the obstinacy of the trouble, are able occasionally, to bring about resorption. The same holds good of the mineral springs containing *Iod.* and *Brom.*, such as Hall, Kreuznach, Wittekind near Halle, Rehme, Kœsen, Reichenhall, Ischl., &c. Besides, we refer to the clinical observations with *Aur.* and *Baryt.*, but also with *Con.*, *Lycopod.*, &c.

NOTE.—It is not so unimportant, as it may seem, to strive in a rational manner for the diminution of hypertrophical glands. Let us be reminded of the consequences of such, frequently hard, glandular swellings. On account of the unavoidable pressure upon the adjacent parts, they may produce results (asthma ; atrophia of the respiratory muscles ; convulsions; paralysis) endangering life which, without proper help, have occasioned painful death. In a like manner we can, *vice versa*, do a great deal of good with curative means so well adapted as ours. Thus we may explain why Spong. cured diseases of the heart of a grave (secondary) character, or why Iod., Brom., Con., &c., softening and resorbing, as they did, occult glandular indurations at a critical locality, removed diseases which, in fact, were to be considered but the sequelæ of a primary glandular affection.

## 2. *Struma.*

The swelling of the thyroid gland is so intimately connected with scrofulosis that formerly the term struma was used for scrofulosis. Goitre is mostly a stationary phenomenon, similar to hypertrophy of the lymphatic glands of the neck, axilla, &c. But its growth, as well as its first unexpected appearance, may make it seem desirable to interfere with it, especially, if dyspnœa or considerable disfigurement results from it. The symptoms of compression depend upon the direction in which the thyroid gland, or single portions thereof, increase in size. A growth anteriorly is most disfiguring, but, at the same time, most favorable as regards general health, especially respiration. On the other hand, disturbances of circulation and respiration appear in consequence of a displacement of the musculi sterno-cleido-mastoidei, in case of lateral or posterior hypertrophy. Disturbances of deglutition and impediments of respiration, if the struma surrounds the œsophagus or trachea in ring form. Enlargements, inferiorly, as far as below the manubrium sterni, are most dangerous.

We distinguish between struma *lymphatica*, a simple enlargement of the glandular knots, and str. *cystica*, an enlargement of the several knots into cysts. Thus, with children cysts may develop of one inch in diameter. A colloid mass (a thickly-fluid, gluey, yellow or brownish liquid) constitutes the contents of the cysts. From globular, tuberous enlargements we may infer struma cystica.

Therapia.—To extirpate strumata for æsthetical reasons is generally condemned. There exists, however, the short-sightedness of recommending painting with Iodine (from six to twelve times, at intervals from three to six days) for the purpose of effecting a cure. The relation of the thyroid gland to the lungs is too important (though not sufficiently understood) to permit without obnoxious consequences, the removal of such hypertrophies (which certainly do not exist without purpose) by external means.

The removal of the pathological products by internal remedies specifically homœopathic is a different matter, however. Among these strictly belong only the *Carbonate of Lime*, which produces strumata, and *Iodium*, of which the same is maintained, and both of which are advantageously combined in the preparation of *Calc. jodata;* besides these, *Iron*, which favors the growth of goitre, may be mentioned here, probably.

Aside from Calc. carb., and Iodium, *Apis* has the name of removing goitre; against struma cystica we should prefer *Calc. carb.*, because, according to experience, other cysts also have given way under its systematic (*i. e.*, temporary discontinuation and administration of the remedy in different dilutions) application.

Spong. and Brom., moreover, in suitable dilutions bring no danger. The term of "Kropf-Schwamm" (goitre-sponge) for Spongia is very properly applied.*

Finally, there is nothing to contraindicate the prudent application of *Kali hydrojod.* (IX.)

### 3. *Chronic Hypertrophy of the Tonsils.*

It may be doubtful whether it is always inherited, as Alfred Vogel thinks, but it is certain that children two years old may be already affected by it. If we inspect the oral cavity

* I can hardly sufficiently recommend the following treatment: Spong. 1, ten drops in two gramm. of Spirit. vin. rectific. Of this morning and evening from two to three drops for several weeks. In chronic cases Spong., in alternation with Brom., Iod., Phosph., especially if dyspnœa, shortness of breathing while walking and ascending stairs result from struma.

of such patients, we see two fleshy plethoric swellings at the side of the uvula; smaller and larger vessels cover them, and single spots are frequently denuded of their common encasing membrane in a manner that makes it appear as if a real almond could be seen behind the defective shell. From the enlargement toward the nose, a nasal voice, snoring and difficult breathing during sleep result, and there is in such children a noticeable disposition to angina, diphtheritis, and membranous croup. Other symptoms of a scrofulous diathesis hardly ever are absent. The enlarged tonsils take position in front of the tuba Eustachii, and occasion hardness of hearing of a higher or less grade and abnormal sounds.

There can be no doubt as to the scrofulous nature of this trouble, for the reason that *Iodium* and its preparations, especially *Calcar. jodata* (Vehsemeyer) affords help. It characterizes itself, moreover, by this, that, though admitting of a certain spontaneous diminution of the glands, in the course of years (in the same manner as inherited strumata heal spontaneously), it yet continues to the age of manhood, and to a later date even. Allopathic physicians praise the efficacy of Cod-liver oil in this affection—a praise that is identical with that of Iodine.

Dupuytren thinks that these glandular swellings, in consequence of the pressure upon the muscles of respiration, atrophy the latter, and thus produce the "chicken-breast" (pectus carinatrum) afterwards. But it is our opinion that, where such tonsilar hypertrophies exist, there is predisposition to tuberculosis ab initio. Hoarseness, shortness of breathing, and easy tiring while speaking, appear in company. If we deprive scrofulosis of the locality chosen by it, *e.g.*, by extirpation or cauterization of the tonsils, or a forced Iodine-treatment, it is likely to be followed by the same sad consequences as are wont to set in in case of treating strumata in the same manner; hence, here even the essence of the disease ought not to be lost sight of over the anatomical lesion.

However, a reasonable administration of the remedies named, as well as of *Calc. phosph.* (jodata?), almost specific in this trouble, and of *Baryt. mur.*, is not excluded.*

* In the Journal des Connaissances Médicales (May 20, 1866), Lambron recommends the mineral sulphur-waters ("en boisson et en douches locales"),

On theoretical grounds, and because this affection, together with ozæna scrofulosa and ophthalmia neonatorum, represents, so to say, the prototype of scrofulosis, two diseases, for which *Mercur. præcipitat. ruber* has proved its efficacy in a brilliant manner, we are inclined to consider this remedy worthy of trial here.

*Kali bichromicum*, a remedy that shows its curative power peculiarly in the most intense and inveterate symptoms of scrofulosis, has likewise produced good results.

Finally, a concentrated extract of the *Folia juglandis*, with which the tonsils were painted, has been used. This means is almost as little deserving of imitation as the gargarisms with Alum and the applications of Nitrate of Silver.

Hardness of hearing, occasioned by hypertrophy of the tonsils, gives way, sometimes, in an amazing manner, upon the administration of *Iod.* and *Brom.* (S. XXX), a fact not explainable without a simultaneous partial resorption of the hypertrophied tissue.

(S. under BARYT., Dr. Zwingenberg's method against hypertrophy of the tonsils.)

---

## *D.*—SCROFULOUS AFFECTIONS OF THE JOINTS AND BONES.

At another place we have called them—rightly or wrongly—the tertiary phenomena of scrofulosis. Other (primary and secondary) scrofulous conditions are wont to precede them, and, no doubt, always do precede them, until the osseous system and skeleton are affected in their turn, as occurrences of much greater significance. As regards our treatise this section is of especial interest to us, in so far as it again offers us a chance for indicting the old school for the inexcusable thoughtlessness which permits it to make use, without the slightest ado whatever, of amputations and operations, where homœopathy treats in the most considerate and conservative manner.

Far from denying the necessity of surgical interference for

---

Luxeuil-Baréges. Dr. Caffe recommends the partial removal of the tonsils (in which case they continue to secrete when food is swallowed).

diagnostic purposes, as well as the removal of pieces of dead sequestrum, the charge of hasty removal of whole limbs by means of saw and knife, has nevertheless to be sustained.

NOTE.—It would be slandering our opponents if, in making the above assertion, not one example observed, at least, stood before our mental eye.

A woman who had suffered for years from caries of the metacarpal bones, and had been advised by every one to have the hand amputated, consulted me last year. Profuse, ichorous suppuration, at several places, exhausted her. The hand was remarkably disfigured by the destructive process.

By means of exclusively homœopathic remedies at long intervals, as well as in more frequent repetitions, I succeeded in relieving the woman to that degree that she could knit, lift cooking utensils, and perform almost all domestic labors with the hand that was considered lost. She received but *Sulph.*, *Calc. carb.*, and *Ferrum jodat.* Her gratitude knew no bounds. The suppuration became confined to a minimum, which worked a favorable change, especially in the disposition of the patient. She became pregnant again, all the while retaining her healthy appearance, gained in flesh, notwithstanding that during pregnancy the suppuration became more profuse and offensive with elimination of small bony fragments.*

## I. SCROFULOUS DISEASES OF THE BONES.

### 1. *Periostitis Scrofulosa*,

(INFLAMMATION OF THE PERIOSTEUM,)

Shows itself as an acute or chronic affection. Yet the chronic form can become acute. Spongy bones are attacked very rarely, but the compact and long ones (tibia, femur, humerus).

The termination in suppuration or ichorous decomposition is preponderantly frequent. Pus is formed between periosteum and bone; abscesses develop in the adjoining soft tissues, which communicate with the pus-foci of the bone, and thus

* In our remarks upon Silic., as one of the most important antiscrofulous remedies, the reader will find a few more such results as described here.

may form a large cavity. Usually the periosteum is detached to a considerable extent, the bone itself necrotizes and ulcerates (caries).

Tuberculous masses appear as products of inflammation.

The pain, dull at the beginning, and worse upon touch, is aggravated by changes of weather and at night. The skin becomes stretched and hard at the diseased spot, until fluctuation and breaking of the abscess take place. Spongy granulations that bleed easily.

The prognosis is unfavorable on account of the frequent transition into necrosis or caries. Its course, to the horror of the patient and his friends, is sometimes exceedingly chronic. A hectic condition may occasion death before complete ulceration and necrotic detachment have taken place.

### 2. *Osteomyelitis*, *Endostitis*.

(INFLAMMATION OF THE MARROW.)

The inflammation of the marrow within the cavum medullare of the cylindrical bones happens with scrofulous subjects, and that very frequently. There exists simultaneously inflammation of the periosteum, and likewise not rarely inflammation of the marrow in the bony network of the short cylindrical bones. All the spaces within the osseous network and the cavum medullare are filled up at the commencement with dark-red marrow, which is rich in blood and cells, sometimes even of a decomposed, puriform character. In its later stages the process is called *osteoporosis*, *osteospongiosis*, *spina ventosa*. Purulent softening and resorption of osseous substance takes place and make the bone appear inflated. In a certain sense we could speak of eccentric hypertrophy, especially, as the simultaneous periostitis deposits lamellose neoplasmata. The joints are apt to remain free from the affection; on this account, and in view of the tuberous swellings in places where enchondroma makes its appearance (metacarpal and metatarsal bones), the affection reminds us of the latter. If those swellings break, numerous but small fistulous openings are formed.

### 3. *Ostitis Scrofulosa.*

(INFLAMMATION OF THE BONE ITSELF.)

A frequent manifestation of scrofula. The spongious bones (short bones of the hand and foot, epiphyses of the long bones—vertebræ) are attacked, especially.

At first, one or more inflammatory foci show themselves. The osseous spaces, which are soon taken possession of by granulations, and show a great richness in cellular structures, are filled up to excess with a fatty-gelatinous liquid; the meshes of the long bones enlarge, bony substance being resorbed by the growth of the granulation (*osteoporosis*).

The bone appears more voluminous at the spot inflamed, though the whole amount of its mass has grown less. Frequently we notice, even if the inflammation reaches the depth of the bone, that the adjacent soft tissues already show forming abscesses.

The tuberculous form of ostitis is frequent among the scrofulous. Several foci form, or a uniform infiltration of the bony substance with a semi-transparent, grayish-yellow, and gelatinous exudation. If separate foci exist, they are surrounded with a kind of capsula which encases, so to say, that exudation, but disappears in consequence of the subsequent changes in the latter. Softening soon takes place; the foci assume a yellowish color; crummy, cheesy elements may be found in a thick-flowing, pappy mass, and in case of a quick enlargement (of the foci), not rarely small bony fragments. In consequence of this process in the bones, caverns are formed which, if several of them run together, make the bones brittle. A cure may be accomplished by resorption of the liquid contents, with simultaneous calcification of the remainder, while in the surroundings thickening of the bony tissue takes place, by which, now and then, encasement is effected. However, perforation and discharge of tuberculous pus with continuation of the process as tuberculous caries are more frequent.

The tuberculous infiltration affects either an entire bone (*e.g.*, a vertebra) or a portion thereof. In the bones, which are permeated by grayish-yellow products of inflammation, yellowish streaks and spots appear which rapidly enlarge, become confluent, and consist of a purulent liquid, intermixed with a crummy mass, which soon assumes the pyonichorous and sanious character. By its influence the bony tissue is destroyed in larger or smaller portions, and may be found sometimes in the ichorous discharge. If the process progresses, it may affect the periosteum, and occasion its ichorous decomposition and destruction.

The terminations of scrofulous ostitis are:

1. Resorption (exceedingly rare).

2. Suppuration with subsequent healing *without transition* into caries. This termination also is rare, if perforation and discharge have taken place. Under the influence of the dyscratic diathesis,

3. Caries, or

4. Necrosis,

follow much oftener.

### *Caries.*

The characteristics of caries consist in this, that it affects spongious bones, usually develops from primary ostitis; progresses from the interior of the bone to its surface (caries centralis), and much more rarely migrates from the periosteum inwardly (caries peripherica). The osseous ulcer "par excellence" is produced, if the carious inflammation attacks a circumscribed spot; for several spots may be affected. The bone may ulcerate at one time in separate portions (C. partialis), at another *in toto* (C. totalis).

Caries develops in this way: the granulations secrete a reddish-brown liquid which, in combination with the decomposing fat-cells and the few pus-corpuscles, produces the ichor with which the spaces of the osseous network are filled. Then atrophia of the osseous partition-walls takes place, in consequence of which the bone thus diseased becomes soft and compressible until it entirely disappears on account of the destruction progressing from layer to layer.

Caries *necrotica* takes place, if portions of the bone, themselves normal, which are adjacent to the carious spots, are deprived of nutrition, die off, and form smaller or larger pieces of sequestrum.

The soft tissues participate the more as the carious process progresses; the connective tissue is attacked by ulceration, especially, where the periosteum is destroyed. Larger or smaller purulent foci and fistulæ form; perforation outwardly, discharge of the carious ichor.

The secretion is mostly thin, of a nauseating disgusting smell (similar to decomposing meat), intermixed with bony particles, or in case of tuberculous caries, with caseous crumbs and flakes (and bony particles). Spongious granulations sprout up around the fistulous opening which frequently cover the entrance and easily bleed upon touch. The ichor often gets to the surface by a circuitous route. The silver probe, which becomes blackened on account of the sulphur-compound of the ichor, feels the diseased bony part rough, uneven, worm-eaten, as it were, and compressible.

If smaller bones, distant from the trunk, are affected by caries, the general health suffers but little.

In case of a cure the atrophy of the bones ceases, the discharge stops, the granulations become more firm and richer in fibres; then ossification and repair of the substance lost start at those granulations, as well as at the adjacent tissue, and especially at the thickened periosteum.

### *Necrosis.*

All the causes and conditions of caries may also produce necrosis. In consequence of undermining the periosteum or membrana medullaris, and of pressure upon the vessels after copious exudations have been deposited, a piece of bone becomes isolated, and dies off. According to the seat and extent, we distinguish likewise between superficial, internal (central), partial, or total necrosis. In contradistinction to the carious process, necrosis affects more the long, cylindrical bones. It is plain, moreover, that the anatomico-physiological peculiarities of the part affected modify scrofulosis, which, in its essence, remains the same always. Hence necrosis appears here, and caries there. In the same manner sclerotitis develops in one case, and a stye in another under the same, *e. g.*, rheumatic influence. But necrosis itself, even, appears to be different according to its seat.

*a.* In central necrosis the isolated piece of bone, deprived of nutrition—the sequestrum—is found to be inclosed in a capsula lined with granulations—death-shrine. From the capsula incasing the sequestrum, openings, varying in number, take their departure, which are also lined with granulations, and lead in an outward direction (*cloacæ*).

The holes in the bones are round or oval, variable in size, and externally surrounded by a wall of granulation; pus issues therefrom as long as the sequestrum is within the capsula, and though they may temporarily heal up, usually break open again soon.

If the sequestrum is removed the cavity is filled with granulations, and forthwith by a granular mass, provided that the general health has not run down too much; and the fistulous sinuses heal up, mostly by leaving cicatricial contractions.

*b.* In superficial necrosis, after periostitis, the sequestrum usually is not incased in a complete capsula; on this account it can be expelled more easily. The canal in which it was imbedded fills up with granulations, and a cicatrix is formed immediately adhering to the bone.

*c.* In necrosis totalis a complete "death-shrine" is likewise but rarely formed; this is pierced, on the contrary, by openings; the soft tissues are traversed by wide and long fistulous sinuses.

*d.* Lastly, the dying off of whole bones takes place occasionally, *e. g.*, in case of scrofulosis at the hand and foot, as sequela of intense ostitis and periostitis. Hence, the sequestrum, consisting of the entire bone, shows traces of inflammation, sometimes is carious, even, in a high degree, osteo-porous, and imbedded in a wide cavern filled with pus and ichor.

If the swelling has broken, or been opened, we reach the dead bone through the opening; in most cases it gives a hard sound upon touch, and feels smooth and firm.

### *Spondylarthrocace.*

#### SCROFULOUS INFLAMMATION OF THE VERTEBRÆ—MALUM POTII, KYPHOSIS PARALYTICA.

In scrofulous children, either spontaneously, or upon some injury, such as a fall, &c., one or more vertebræ become inflamed often, with inclination to ulcerous destruction of the bone (as central caries); the affection usually sets in in form of infiltrated tuberculosis. If caverns have formed by softening of the tuberculous masses, and the vertebra cannot resist any longer the weight of the parts above it, curving in of the vertebræ takes place. The curvature mostly takes place posteriorly (Kyphosis, Malum Pottii), but is combined with lateral curvature also (Skoliosis, Kyphosis skoliotica). The symptoms of an affection of the spinal marrow, dependent thereupon, are not always of a grave character.

Another sequela we observe in the so-called metastatic abscesses (which extend mostly along the anterior side of the spinal column, and appear at the groin or small pelvis). Perforation with discharge into the spinal canal is rare. The quality of the pus corresponds to its origin; it is thin, ichorous, intermixed with decomposed tuberculous masses and osseous fragments and remnants of ligaments; has an offensive smell, and discolors the probe, &c.

Pains, either fixed or migratory, are the first symptom. Afterwards loss of appetite, febrile attacks, sleeplessness, decrease of mental capacity. The curvature appears at a later date, and mostly gradually.

According to the seat of the affection we speak of spondylarthrocace thoracica, cervicalis (angina Hippocratis), lumbalis, and sacralis.

THERAPIA.—The acute stages of periostitis may be met with *Aconit.* and *Bellad.*, yet *Mercur.*, above all, seems to be able to effect resorption and amelioration of the intense nocturnal pains (LXXXV). *Mercur.* and *Phosph.* produce necrosis, and both have done excellent service in its homœopathic treatment. The excessive formation of pus, and the consumption of strength therewith connected, may be prevented by injections of *Iodine.* Though *Aurum* is said to correspond more to syphilitic necrosis, yet we know that scrofulous ozæna, depending upon bony ulceration of the nose, is also cured by *Aurum;* more frequently, however, by *Hydr. præc. rubr.* From the curative influence of the remedies mentioned upon the carious and necrotic process, the cures of some cases of hardness of hearing, and many results in dental practice, may be explained. *However*, SILICEA *has been and remains the most important remedy in the treatment of (scrofulous) diseases of the bones; no other drug so hastens the elimination of the dead bony particles (to the largest piece of sequestrum) necessary for a cure.*

*Caustic.*, which may also be applied externally as injection, or in the form of compresses and pledgets, as has been described above, removes the burning pains often very troublesome in the neighborhood of the fistulous openings of carious affections.

*Calcar.* and *Sulph.*, by improving the general constitution, are surely able to exert a favorable influence upon the course of caries or necrosis, though they do not exert the direct influence that *Silic.* does. The same is true of *Hep. sulph. calc.* and *Baryt.* (S. XVIII).

Of the metastatic abscesses, such as occur in malum Pottii, those only ought to be opened (subcutaneously) the breaking of which is to be regarded as unavoidable at any rate. Here, also, *Iodine* injections may be used afterwards, for the purpose of averting the appearance of hectic fever (Jousset). The action of *Calc. carb.* in spondylarthrocace is plainly visible from Case XLVII.

## II. SCROFULOUS INFLAMMATIONS OF THE JOINTS.

According as the inflammation takes its departure, either from the osseous portion or from the synovial membrane lining the joint, we observe two pathological processes entirely different from each other. In the former case, *arthrocace;* in the latter, *Tumor albus*, or the *fungous* inflammation.

Displacement of the epiphyses, by a disturbance of the apparatus holding the parts together, may easily occur.

Although any synovial membrane may be affected, and give rise to fungous inflammation, and every end of the bone that helps to form a joint may lead to arthrocace, yet the most favored seat of the latter is the hip-joint, and of the former the knee-joint; and we select, therefore, *coxarthrocace*, as representative of the one class of scrofulous inflammation of the joints, and *tumor albus genu* of the other.

### *The Scrofulous Inflammation of the Hip-Joint.*

COXITIS SCROFULOSA; COXARTHROCACE; COXALGIA MORBUS COXARUM; LUXATIO SPONTANEA.

This affection belongs to those scrofulous troubles which are apt to show themselves during the second period of dentition.

1. *Acute Course.*—Starting at the caput femoris, it is, in acute cases, accompanied by the most intense pain at the inside of the thigh down to the knee, increasing upon touch or use of the joint. Sleep is disturbed. Exhausting, febrile motions. The thigh is somewhat adduced inwardly. The buttock swollen. Its fold stands lower. The affected extremity appears longer or shorter. The termination in suppuration is accompanied by the formation of abscesses in the neighborhood of the joint which communicate with the latter. In consequence of the consumption of a portion of the femoral head a disturbance in space takes place, and escape of the head out of the acetabulum. Hectic fever and pyæmia lead to fatal termination. In rare cases only the suppuration diminishes, portions of the bone are detached, and the openings of the abscesses close up.

2. *Chronic Course.*—Insignificant dragging of the extremity in walking; easy tiring and complaints of weakness and stiffness of the leg as well as unsteady gait indicate the beginning disease. The vague, insignificant pain running down the leg resembles the rheumatic. It is present mostly in the morning, and sometimes in the evening accompanied by febrile symptoms. There is hardly anything abnormal in the hip-joint; yet, the diseased extremity when lifted up, is apt to assume the position mentioned above (drawing up of the leg with foot inverted). These conditions, with intermissions may exist for months and years even.

If the disease exacerbates, the characteristic pain in the *knee* appears which, however, does not aggravate upon touch or motion, and which some have attempted to explain by irritation of the nervous obturatorius or saphenus int. In stooping the patients use the healthy knee and keep the diseased leg stiff. Limping is occasioned. In sitting also, the body rests upon the healthy hip. In walking the point of the foot of the diseased extremity touches the floor. As regards the question, agitated for a good while, whether shortening or elongation of the diseased extremity takes place, this much is settled now, that neither the one nor the other exists, but such an elongation or shortening takes place apparently* only, on account of a sinking down, or rising of one side of the pelvis (displacement upwardly with subsequent spinal curvature). Hence, those theories, according to which the (apparent) shortening is said to arise from muscular strain and contraction which were to press the femoral head against the acetabulum; or, according to which, on the other hand, the head was to be pressed downwardly in consequence of effusions, exudations, &c., to produce the (apparent) elongation, must be abandoned forever.

In this, so to say, second stage even, resorption, *i.e.*, a cure, is possible. If not, the suppuration increases after previous swelling, redness, fluctuation, metastatic abscesses into the knee-joint and still lower down; finally, on account of carious destruction of the femoral head and decrease of its size; disproportion with regard to the acetabulum, and *real*, not apparent elongation or shortening and spontaneous luxation occur. The femoral head escapes mostly posteriorly, and upon the upper external surface of the os ilei, rarely into the foramen obturatorium, or upon the horizontal portion of the os pubis. Exceptionally the decayed femoral head has been discharged through a fistulous opening. If the ligamentum capsulare is perforated by pus, the perforation takes place mostly at its posterior or inferior portion. Not unfrequently we observe that the pus escapes from the cavity of the joint at the point of communication with the bursa mucosa subcutanea beneath the musculus ilio-psoas into the latter, and thence into the pelvic cavity, though the pus may also get into the pelvic cavity by perforating the os ilei at the point

* In proof thereof the following modus operandi has been proposed: Both spinæ anteriores superiores of the patient, who is in a lying position, are brought into a line as straight as possible; upon this a second straight line is drawn, starting at the processus xiphoideus sterni. Then we try to bring both extremities in precisely the same position, and measure with a rule of solid material from the spina to the condyl. int. tibiæ and malleolus int.

of the gluteal muscles. The fistulous openings formed by the perforation of the skin are mostly surrounded by spongious and easily-bleeding granulations which rise above the level of the skin.

Extensive cutaneous and subcutaneous ulcers in the neighborhood of the point of perforation are not of rare occurrence.

THERAPIA.—In *Rhus* and *Silicea* we possess two remedies which, according to experience, have cured cases of coxarthrocace not too far developed (S. XCV, CII, CCV, CXIII). But *Silic.* would be preferable to other remedies in the most desperate cases of coxarthrocace, even; for the malignity of the trouble could be owing only to a deeper affection of the bones, the very domain of *Silicea. Iodium* and its preparations require caution, though we shall report at another place an interesting cure with *Ol. jec. aselli.* (LXVII). After Silicea; *Calc.* and also *Sulph.* have to be given frequently, after which fresh doses of Silicea evince a more penetrating effect. A change in the dose (between 30th and 3d), and a steady, slow action of the remedy (one dose daily, at the highest) secure a good result.

## *The Scrofulous Inflammation of the Knee-Joint.*

### TUMOR ALBUS GENU; GONARTHROCACE; GONALGIA, WHITE SWELLING AT THE KNEE.

The affection has been counted among the white swellings for the reason that the synovial membrane is the terminating point of the inflammation more frequently than the condyli and ligaments. Its course, as in similar cases, may be exceedingly acute, even suddenly lethal, as well as slow and dragging.

Its pathological picture is self-constructing, so to say, since the usual symptoms of inflammation, redness, heat, swelling, stiffness, functional disturbance of the part and pain manifest themselves. At the beginning the knee is bent. If it comes to suppuration, the pus discharges now above the knee, now burrows toward the malleoli of the leg, and may appear at any place (though not anteriorly). In consequence of caries of the bones, dislocation of the lower leg may take place.

*Terminations:* cure in every stage of the disease; continuous stiffness of the knee, produced by spurious or genuine anchylosis; hence, tendinous adhesions of the connective tissue, or osseous adhesions. In case of fatal termination it is preceded by œdematous swelling and very copious, ichorous discharge.

THERAPIA.—The chronic white swelling of the knee is very obstinate, though very good results may be obtained by *Calcar.* and *Silic.* According to Kallenbach's experience, the pressing, stitching pain, intermitting at rest and during the night, is bearable, if the case corresponds to *Calc. carb.* In the reverse case, *Baryt. carb.* is said to be preferable.

Mineral springs (Teplitz) ought also not to be undervalued. Sulphur springs, as well as sand-baths, the value of which is more and more appreciated nowadays, deserve our full confidence. The more the organism is attacked in its inmost parts by the scrofulous process, as is the case in all affections of the bones and joints, the more we must endeavor to produce a more energetic exchange of matter and a more efficient expulsion of organic cinders by an increased activity of the peripheric organs, *i. e.*, of the skin in our case; and this is accomplished by the full bath, aside from the possibility of thus permitting the specific remedy to act upon the body upon an extent of surface as great as possible. Among the cures by *Silic.*, a case is also mentioned in which decoctions of grass-seed, applied externally, were of essential benefit. We gladly notice such observations, because they all evince the purpose to allow the really active agent (here Silic.), to exhibit its effect by breaking up the cohesion of its particles to a considerable extent.

Besides Silicea, Calcar., Baryt., and the preparations of Sulphur; *Rhus*, *Caustic.*, *Ferrum*, *Kali*, *Merc.*, and *Phos.*, as well as *Iodium*, in low dilutions, may be recommended, most of which have already proved their efficacy by clinical tests.

Heyne prefers Calcar. *phos.* to Calc. carb. in tumor albus. The cure of a scrofulous inflammation of the knee-joint we shall report at another place. See Case LI.

# III.

## THE MOST APPROVED REMEDIES AGAINST SCROFULA.

---

THE rationality of the antiscrofulous treatment is certainly decisive as regards the prognosis and eventuality of relapses. Orthodox allopathic treatment offers the worst guarantees. By its mania forthwith to bleed in every case of hyperæmia and trifling pain, it contributes to the derangement of the bodily constitution. The blood, already predisposed to dropsy, is made still more watery.*

Moreover, by its anointing and exsiccating method (using zinc, lead, and mercurial salves, astringent injections, &c.), it induces the *vis medicatrix naturæ*, aiming at the expulsion of the inimical matter, again to transfer those causes, imponderable though they be, yet morbific in their action, to internal organs. For this very reason we can indorse only that portion of the therapeutics of allopathic authorities which dwells upon general hygienic rules, and is, for the greatest part, of a purely prophylactic nature.

Self-evidently, the homœopathic physician will not oppose the recommendation of pure air, proper strengthening and concentrated food, the culture of the skin as far as it can possibly go, nor a cautious hardening of the body, if the disease has not, as yet, progressed too far. An exclusively vegetable diet is to be forbidden from the very fact that the scrofulous represent the vegetable type of man in an abnormal manner,

---

* It is certain that in the scrofulous an anomaly exists in the proportion between the solid and liquid organic parts; and this anomaly, as Portal has shown, exists, in all probability, at the expense of the red parts of the blood, or in favor of its serous portion.

and live a life that is already too vegetative. Hence, an animal diet has to be ordered at the same time. Everything favoring the production of acidity (eating of too much fruit),* very salty, also sweet (cane sugar), highly seasoned and fat food, has to be avoided. In short, the diet ought not, as a general thing, to be irritating.

As already mentioned, pure, dry, and warm air, is also necessary for a radical removal of scrofulous affections. Warm clothing prevents the recession of sweat. Dancing, fencing, hunting, riding on horseback, swimming, working in the field or garden, would, no doubt, be very risky undertakings, since in all such exercises the body is thrown into a profuse sweat. Gymnastic exercises, rationally conducted, seem most beneficial.

Scrofulous residents are found but rarely near the ocean. Hence the benefit of residing near the sea might be inferred *a priori*. Let us add to this that, according to experience, sea-baths have rendered most excellent service in removing the scrofulous habitus. The percentage of Iod., Brom., Natr. mur., &c., contained in sea-water, no doubt explains this effect. Sea-air alone contributes essentially to an increase of appetite. Tissot, Cullen, Borden, and others, place especial value in therapeutic aid. Here belong also, the baths of Barêges, Plombières, Mont d'Or, as well as our baths in the North and Baltic Seas.

There exist different views,† however, as regards the value of milk. Baillon, Richard, &c., recommend the milk of asses. Others believe that all milk does harm. The idea that by a strengthening regimen, living in the country, &c., the digestive organs can be so strengthened as to bear milk is, probably correct. Then, it certainly becomes and remains a very

* I frequently observed an increase of scrofulous exanthemata and aggravation of scrofulous ophthalmia from eating cherries or prunes, and after the abuse of apples and apple-butter.

† Thus Alfred Vogel, the celebrated physician of diseases of children, whom we have already quoted several times, says with regard to the diet of rhachitic children: "Cow's milk is the best food for children up to the age of three years. It cannot be compensated by any other, and ought to be given in quantities as large as possible." Dr. Weil, on the contrary, says: "In rhachitis milk must be entirely dispensed with, because by the use of it the bones grow softer and softer."

valuable article of food which is to be estimated more highly, since, as is well known, all the constituents of the blood may also be found in the milk.

Scrofulous children frequently suffer from diarrhœa. In such cases milk-diet ought to be abandoned for a time. Salep and arrowroot hardly answer as substitutes; even Liebig's celebrated soup does not always agree with children. Grits and barley-water, when they are borne well, are not nutritious enough. On the contrary chicken broth prepared from an old chicken with soft-boiled farina, is to be greatly recommended, and may be taken as a substitute for milk for a week and longer. Goat's milk is tried too little, as yet, where cow's milk is not well borne. We hear the objection also, that goat's milk is too fat; yet, the capricious stomach, in such cases, just requires fat, in a similar manner, as there is often an unexpected tolerance of Cod-liver oil. Besides I have ordered the goat's milk to be given warm as it is drawn from the bag, and imagine that I have saved more than one child by this means.

Finally, we mention acorn coffee as a dietetic aid of importance. I heard from trustworthy mothers that their weakly children had begun to walk only since they had been given acorn coffee. This is easily explained, if we remind ourselves of the roborant and tonic property of this drink which contains tannin.

Dr. Weil, no doubt, was supported by similar experiences, since he orders the following regimen for weakly, scrofulous, and rhachitic children.

For breakfast: two cupfuls of acorn coffee, or of homœop. coffee (prepared of half an ounce thereof) with the addition of some sugar and a little milk.

For luncheon, he recommends finely scraped (raw) veal or beef spread over a piece of twist.

For dinner: beef tea, lean, roasted meat, a few vegetables, stewed fruit, wheat bread, light desserts (prepared of eggs).

For supper: soup prepared of farina or grits.

The use of good and pure malt-beer is very beneficial to such children.*

---

* Anleitung zur diaetetischen Krankenpflege von Dr. med. Weil, S. 161. Gotha, 1869.

Bathing in water containing Iod. and Brom., still approaches to homœopathic ideas; though we have accustomed ourselves to set up strict indications for such aids. The same holds good of Cod-liver oil, of which we shall speak anon. However, we will here mention that authors of name deem it indispensable in rhachitis.

The following recommendations in allopathic textbooks we consider to evince but little rationality:

"Several vegetable substances, such as Dulcam., Sarsapar., Cicuta, Folia jugl., &c," as if one and the same antiscrofulous principle were contained in all of them. How differently the physician thinks and judges who treats according to the strictest symptomatic similarity, and is guided by the Mat. Med. PURA. He knows that among the "several vegetable substances" the one corresponds only to this, the other to that pathological complex, diseased individual and disease-stage. In place of arbitrariness a necessary law exists for him.

It is remarkable, notwithstanding, that as regards the most sovereign antiscrofulosa, both schools join hands unconsciously. Who would wish to deny that Cicuta, in fact, is one of our foremost (antiscrofulous) remedies (I refer only to blepharitis cil., scroful.). Hufeland concedes to Baryt. mur. one of the first places among the exceedingly few antiscrofulosa which he accepts, and our homœopathic literature contains the most remarkable cures of intense scrofulosis by Baryt. mur. What important parts do Iod., Ferrum, and the compounds of both; the mercurialia and ammonia preparations, play here as well as there. Aside from these, however, we possess a sufficient number of peculiar remedies. For, of what value are Arsen., the Carbonate of Lime, Sulph., and Nitri acid., to traditional medicine?

Let us now proceed to the valuation of the several antiscrofulosa. We intended at first to arrange them in a manner differing from a mere alphabetical enumeration; yet, no essential gain would result therefrom for practice. If we divide, for example, the antiscrofulosa into such as are of organic or inorganic nature, we should have to separate Graphit. from Carb. veg., and the latter again from Carb. anim., though all three of them have many phenomena in common, *e.g.*, their relations to the glands; moreover, for the sake of consistency, we should have to separate Lycopod. from Calc. carb., and to place the former in the category in which Calendula, Viola tricol., Euphrasia, &c., belong. And where should we speak of Apis which we cannot pass over in silence, entirely; though its curative power in scrofulous ophthalmia and its result (opacity of the cornea) has been doubted, or is not proved, at least, as is that of Acid. nitri., Calcar. carb., &c.

For this reason let us not sacrifice to the mania for classification, the only principle which can engage our consideration regarding the comparison of the various medicinal substances, *i.e.*, the principle of the physiological proving. And here we find that remedies of the organic world may bear similar relations to the same organs as do remedies of the inorganic; hence, that in therapeutics they call for a similar application.

We have given the several reports of cures mostly verbatim, because a short *résumé*, no matter how good a survey it may offer, always lacks the agreeable impression of immediate, personal experience. It is more profitable, if we participate in the subjective impressions of the author in the course of a clinical report; if we feel with him his troubles, and finally enjoy with him the favorable termination.

Finally, we have interfused, here and there, in a somewhat independent manner, practical remarks and hints of the most various observers, and hope that every one—notwithstanding he may miss therein, perhaps, organic connection—will judge for himself and, by the aid of experiences already gained for himself, gain in surety and ease, successfully to grapple with the host of scrofulous diseases.

## ACIDUM NITRI.

### GENERALITIES.

*Acid. nitri* is homœopathically specific in all aphthous ulcers of the mouth, in phlyctænæ of the cornea developing into superficial ulcers; inflammations of the connective tissue of the inner canthus (*ægilops*), terminating in suppuration and subsequent ulceration; in superficial and offensive ulcers accompanying balanorrhœa.

Moreover, in many cases of common scrofulous ophthalmia

(ophthal. pustul., herpes conjunctivæ, Ruete), especially in the later stages, at the height of the inflammation, and after Calcar. carb. has been given in vain.

Most of my colleagues will admit that those cases of scrofulous ophthalmia sometimes belong among the most tedious, because most obstinate objects of cure existing. Merc., Arsen., Hepar., Lycopod., Conium, and Heaven knows what else, are tried, with and without the patience of the physician and patient, and—fail. However, in many such cases, we will yet be rewarded upon the administration of *Acid. nitri.**

Aside from scrofulous ophthalmia, which is not dangerous, but often very obstinate, *Acid. nitri* is indispensable in ophth. neonat., a fact from which we may, probably, infer very correctly the scrofulous nature of this disease; or we may say that, in both cases, one and the same morbid diathesis exists, which finds its curative simile in *Acid. nitri.*†

It remains but to point to the following symptoms of *Acid. nitri*, as recorded in the M. M. P., the complex of which presents a characteristic picture of scrofulous ophthalmia:

"Pressing in the eyes as from sand, in the outer canthi; winking; great sensitiveness to light; stitches and itching in the eyes; smarting and burning; redness of the white; inflammation of the conjunctiva; swelling of the lids; spots upon the cornea; watering of the eyes; acrid humor; agglutination; difficult opening of the lids in the morning; photophobia; obscurity of sight; the right eye becomes obscure; objects appear dark; mist before the eyes; myopia."

The symptoms of *Nitr. ac.*, enumerated under the head of "Ears and Nose," likewise indicate that we possess in this remedy a true antiscrofulosum, and practice has long ago confirmed this supposition in a brilliant manner. It has proved efficacious in hardness of hearing (afterwards Petroleum).

---

* Six drops of the 3d dil. in 60 grammes of water, morning and evening a teaspoonful.

† Ten drops of Acid. nitri 1 or 2, in a saucerful of water; compresses moistened therewith, and applied to the eyes; over the compresses a cloth for protection; the dry compresses to be removed.

## CLINIQUE.

### 1. (I.) *Ophthalmia Scrofulosa.*

L. W., æt. 4, for a year has suffered from scrofulous ophthalmia. The lids of the right eye are red and swollen; vessels of the eye injected, the cornea opaque, especially below the pupil; photophobia; the eye waters, especially when looking into the light; lids are agglutinated in the morning, and itch; from the right nasal opening a watery discharge; a nodulous eruption at the buttocks; crusts and soreness behind the ears. The trouble began with a purulent, offensive tinea capitis et faciei.

Sulph., Bellad., Calcar., Euphras. effected nothing. Puls. 12, alternated every fourth day with *Ac. nitr.* 12, occasioned a considerable aggravation, upon which improvement followed so rapidly, however, that this chronic trouble was completely removed within twenty days. (Erfahrungen aus der Praxis v. Haustein, A. H. Z., 39, 10.)

### 2. (II.) *Blepharitis Phlegmonosa.*

(Observation of my own, A. H. Z., 69, 13.)

The daughter of the stonemason G., æt. 5, has been treated allopathically for six days, until the increasing aggravation has induced the parents to abandon this treatment. There existed a phlegmonous inflammation of the upper, and afterwards of the lower lid; the skin of the lid discolored, swelling of the connective tissue considerable, so that the bulbus could not be seen; the ciliary glands secrete a gluey humor, which mixes with the tears discharged in profusion; the child had fever, was very restless, and the whole affection made an unfavorable impression.

Mercur. viv. 3. (Cotton to the swollen lid.)

December 7th (*i. e.*, the day following). The swelling has gone down remarkably. Less pain. Skin less discolored. Better in general.

One dose of Mercur.

Dec. 9th, without any cause (known) the lower lid is inflamed again and swollen. Bellad. 12, every two hours.

Dec. 10th. More satisfactory state of things. Yet the condition remained oscillating, notwithstanding Bellad. given in alternation with Sulph.

In the surrounding of the eye, purulent-crusty exanthemata formed which *bled easily.* This symptom led us to give *Acid. nitri* 9th dil., every two hours. *The effect was surprising.* From this time on improvement was steady and rapid.

## APIS.

### GENERALITIES.

Dr. Genzke, of Buetzow, aside from an increased frequency of the pulse, which he rightly ascribes in part to the action of the alcohol, observed *obscuration of sight* from the continued use, and large doses of Apis-tincture. At the conjunctiva and membrana nictitans (of the dog experimented upon) distinct vascular injections showed themselves, on account of which the cornea assumed a smoky appearance, and the eyelids were agglutinated in the morning by the mucus secreted. These symptoms continued during the remainder of the proving, and soon disappeared after its termination (N. Z. f. h. Kl., 5, 23).

These are facts. On the other hand, there is scarcely any remedy in the application of which one may deceive himself more than in that of Apis (see, also, Bolle's popul. Zeitschrift, Jahrg., 1866, 1 and 2).

Dr. Genzke noticed, further, that *Apis* (2d dil.) produced satisfactory results in rheumatic, catarrhal, and scrofulous ophthalmia. It acted splendidly in young persons, and especially in acute cases. In older persons and in inveterate cases the effect was but palliative or naught. (In both of the latter conditions we would direct the attention to *Euphrasia* internally and externally.)

Dr. Battmann, of Grossenhain, has observed of *Apis* 2— other remedies had been given in vain previously — several times a very surprising effect in inflammation of the conjunctiva palpebrarum, scleroticæ and corneæ, with vesicles or small ulcers, and infiltrated vascular nets around them, accompanied by photophobia, often of a very high grade, watering of the eyes, pressing and smarting pain. B., for his dilution, used a mother-tincture prepared of three bees, which were mashed in one drachm of diluted alcohol. (N. Z. f. h. Kl., iv, 4).

Dr. Paulson obtained good results with Apis in struma (*Apis* 15th and 30th) (A. H. Z., 72, 22). A remedy that accomplishes results in this direction surely deserves to be counted rightfully among the antiscrofulosa. The cures, moreover, were obtained in individuals who had passed childhood long ago, and of whom no other symptoms of scrofulosis are mentioned.

### CLINIQUE.

#### 1. (III.) *Ophthalmia Scrofulosa.*

A girl, aged thirteen years, who for nearly a year had been suffering from an inflammatory affection of the right eye — a condition which, in spite of former medical treatment, and especially within three months, became so aggravated gradually that the *power of sight was totally annulled*, and the patient was tortured by severe pains appearing in paroxysms, exhibited the following pathological picture: Conjunctiva inflamed in its entire extent; redness more saturated at the outer canthus. From this point a so-called "*scrofulo-vascular ribbon*" departs, which threatens to develop into a pterygium, and sufficiently explains the complete disturbance of the power of sight. On examination of the eye a stream of tears gushes out. Great photophobia; pain on opening the eye; increased secretion of mucus. Agglutination of the lids in the morning. The nose of the child considerably swollen without being inflamed.

Every evening one dose of the 2d dil. of the bee-tincture. Within fourteen days a considerable improvement had set in; the conjunctivitis had nearly disappeared, the pseudo-membranes had become thinner, and had redrawn from the cornea; an opacity still remained upon the latter which did not permit of complete sight. Pain, flow of tears, agglutination of the lids had entirely disappeared. Four weeks afterwards the same prescription, after which the trouble could be considered as entirely removed, with the exception of a nebulous spot upon the cornea at the pupillary edge.

The power of sight is completely restored. The opacity gave way rapidly upon the use of *Aurum* 3 (one dose every other evening).

Dr. Genzke, to whom we are indebted for this report, adds with good reason: This removal, rapid and mild as it is, of a firmly-rooted disease of the eye, allows of no comparison with the treatment of allopathic oculists who, in such a case, undertake at first to combat it by local applications of caustic, or so-called astringent remedies; and since they almost always fail in this, proceed with an operation which, in the most favorable case even, too often only leaves behind a permanent opacity of the cornea (N. Z. f. h. Kl., 5, 34).

### 2. (IV.) *Ophthalmia Scrofulosa.*

Dr. Bolle recommends *Apis* against scrofulous diseases of the eye. He reports (A. H. Z., 52, 6) two interesting cures. *Apis* 1,* was given, and in the one case an obstinate photophobia removed, in the other total blindness, *i. e.*, complete opacity of the cornea in front of the pupil. Even a *scabious* eruption at the neck appeared upon the girl, one year old, after six powders (morning and evening one powder). She had been afflicted previously with genuine itch.

Regarding these results, Dr. Gerster remarks that we ought to be cautious in judging of the influence of such remedies. His words deserve to be quoted here.†

### 3. (V.) *Struma.*

A young lady had an enlargement of the thyroid gland.

---

* Six grains of Apis to one and a half drachm of Alcohol. Globules wetted with this tincture.

† Without doubting in the slightest the highly praised curative action of Apis against scrofulous ophthalmia, and especially against photophobia of scrofulous children, I beg to be permitted the remark that such troubles frequently make remissions, intermissions, exacerbations, and metastases with or without the use of remedies. The aural discharge, facial and cranial eruptions, for instance, disappear, and in their place inflammations of the ocular membranes, phlyctænæ, photophobia, &c., appear; or the aural disease ceases, and otorrhœa, tinea faciei, crusta lactea, swelling of the cervical glands, flowing coryza, &c., set in. Since scrofulous affections of the eye are not a local disease but the expression of a constitutional anomaly, relapses are avoided most surely, if we succeed in removing as much as possible the fundamental trouble by the aid of nature or art.

8

*Iod.*, *Calc. carb.*, and *Rhus* effected nothing; *Apis* 15 and 30. The swelling of the size of a goose-egg has disappeared within fourteen days. Patient was somewhat amenorrhœic during the time of her illness.

4. (VI.) *Struma.*

Mrs. G., æt. 35, suffered every eight days from profuse uterine hemorrhage. She was pale, and could scarcely walk; the right lung hepatized; violent cough morning and evening, with yellowish-gray expectoration; at the same time she was afflicted with goitre. *Calc. carb.* and *Natr. mur.* entirely cured the patient; the goitre only, though somewhat smaller, still existed. After *Apis* 3, within three weeks, no decrease of the struma; after *Apis* 30, morning and evening four globules, the enlargement disappeared gradually.

5. (VII.) *Struma.*

Mrs. L., æt. 43, in climacteric years. Menses irregular. Pain in the left and right ovary; large struma, with difficulty of breathing. *Apis* 15, six globules morning and evening, completely cured the struma within fourteen days (the remaining symptoms were cured by *Sepia*) (Western Hom. Observer, July 15th, 1865).

## ARSENICUM.

### GENERALITIES.

*Arsen.* does not act directly or specifically upon the morbid product, as an antiparasitic, as it were, but upon the healthy tissue, the vital energy of which it increases, and which it enables to resist the inroad of the pathological element. Restoring general health, it becomes one of the surest remedies to counteract the development of neoplasmata. This occurs in the *scrofulides* which aggravate the scrofula-cachexia, and in superficial and deep suppurations, pulmonary catarrhs, accompanied by profuse, offensive secretion, fever, *emaciation*, and *marasmus;* in *parasitismus*, in the course of convalescences dragging out for a long time; finally in *tubercle.* Its efficacy in cancer is still illusory, though we possess several observations not to be underrated in this direction also.*

With *Arsenic* we find, as a rule, *a check of the organic activity, similar to paralysis;* on the other hand, inclination to profuse secretions chemically alienated (Northoff, d. Hom., 33, 108).

"It is always," says a third author, "the ulcerative process, and especially the ulcerative process inclining to atonia and gangrenescence which succumbs to the curative power of *Arsenic*. Against phagedenic impetigo and herpetic ulcers, *Arsen.* has often been recommended" (Dr. Frank, Osterode, A. H. Z., 31, 23).

From Rueckert's "attempts at utilizing the curative material obtained ab usu in morbis," we quote the following indications: Nasal openings, corners of the mouth and anus red and sore; ulcers at the nostrils; annoying burning; sensation of paralysis of the tongue; unquenchable thirst; intense burning at the anus; coryza, acrid, corroding the upper lip; violent burning beneath the skin (in bed); chronic eruptions; tinea capitis in which *Arsen.* proved itself curative, predominantly showed pustules and vesicles containing a purulent liquid—ulcers discharging a thick, greenish, and offensive ichor—itching *violently*, burning, worse at night; better from warmth, worse from cold air. Small pustular elevations resembling scabies burst, and the corroding liquid forms phagedenic ulcers. Phagedenic bullæ at the soles of the feet, and painful burning over the entire ulcerating surface.

### CLINIQUE.

In cases of scrofulous ophthalmia, *Arsenic* has produced the following results (Z. f. h. Kl., 2, 20):

#### 1. (VIII.) *Ophthalmia Scrofulosa.*

A girl, æt. 20, with opacities upon the cornea from former inflammations suffered from scrofulous ophthalmia of the right eye and lids. Pain at the edge of the cornea; a phlyctæna developing, photophobia, flow of tears.

* Die Heilsamkeit des Antimon-Arseniks gegen Lungenemphysem. v. Dr. Payr in Wuerzburg (A. H. Z., 79, 15).

*Bellad.* 3; cure within three days. A relapse was cured by *Bellad.* within four days, and the remaining flow of tears by *Arsen.* 6.

2. (IX.) *Ophthalmia Scrofulosa.*

A girl, æt. 12, for three weeks suffered from Ophth. scrof. of the left eye with two ulcers on the cornea. Shooting pains. Flow of tears. *Bellad.* 3 without effect. *Arsen.* 3; cure within twenty-three days.

3. (X[a].) *Ophthalmia Scrofulosa.*

A woman, æt. 27, frequently suffering from styes, for the space of four months is affected with scrofulous ophthalmia of the left eye with pricking pain; ulcers on the cornea, photophobia, flow of tears. *Ars.* 12 improved her rapidly, and cured within sixteen days.

Note.—The affections of the eyes cured by *Arsen.* are characterized, according to Dr. Gauwerky, by burning pains and soreness of the inner surface of the lid, obscurity of sight, and amelioration from warmth; spots and ulcers on the cornea, and acrid, corroding tears (9. Jahresvers. d. hom Aerzte Rheinlands und Westphalens, 31. Juli, 1856).

4. (X[b].) *Scrofulous Blennorrhœa of the Eye.*

Dr. John Weber, of Brilon (A. H. Z., 39, 9, 1), cured an intensely itching crusta lactea (in a fleshy girl, six months old), by *Arsen.* 30. The eyes were entirely closed by the swelling, and between the lids an acrid matter oozed out corroding everything around. The child rubbed its head and face almost constantly, and the parents feared that she would become blind.

He also cured a similar tinea by *Arsen.* and several others by *Rhus.*

5. (XI.) *Abdominal Scrofula, Atrophia Infantum.*

In order to give an instructive illustration in which cases *Arsen.* is of extraordinary efficacy, we quote the following clinical observation of Kafka (N. Z. f. h. Kl., 2, 1).

*Atrophia in consequence of Chronic Intestinal Catarrh.*

A boy, æt. 2, had already been affected by diarrhœa for six months. All professional and non-professional means used against it, remained without any result. I was consulted December 9th, 1853, and found the boy emaciated to the highest degree, pale, like a corpse, of withered and senile features. The eyes rolled about wildly in their deep sockets, animatedly following every word and motion of mine and those surrounding. His thirst was not to be quenched; every five or six seconds he asked for a drink. Appetite tolerably keen, yet as soon as food is taken, rumbling in the abdomen sets in, and from four to six fluid, painless stools of an excessively nauseating and cadaverous smell follow each other in quick succession. Their number within twenty-four hours, I was told, approached to from 16 to 20. The abdomen is distended meteoristically, and gives a clear, tympanitic sound at all points with the exception of the region of the liver and spleen, where percussion proves a considerable organic enlargement. Nasal openings, mouth and anus red and sore; dentition has nearly terminated; worms were never passed.

Upon the use of *Arsen.* 6 (10 drops in half pint of water), two teaspoonfuls every two hours, the child was completely convalescent within four weeks.

NOTE.—Although Kafka does not say that the child was scrofulous; leaning upon considerable experience, I yet may maintain that scrofulous children, affected by such chronic diarrhœæ, endangering life, are exceedingly well served by *Arsen.* The 6th dilution has proved itself to me also, the most effective. It is very important not to confound the indications for *Arsen.* with those of *Carb. veg.*

In the N. Z. f. h. Kl., 4, 20, we read of very interesting cures by *Arsen.*, obtained by Dr. Eidherr, of Vienna, in atrophia infantum.

In those cases in which *intermitting* fever, hot head and hands and a disturbance of the process of nutrition plainly manifested themselves, he gave *Arsen.* 15, and followed it up by *Calc. carb.*, if the intermitting fever had disappeared, the children became more lively, and looked better, but the diarrhœic green stools, hardness and tenderness of the abdomen remained.

6. (XII.) *Abdominal Scrofula*, *Atrophia Infantum.*

Harriet B., æt. 1½, a miserable child, emaciated to a skeleton, with a large, distended abdomen, and thin legs, upon which the muscles hung down like old rags, the skin of the whole body shrivelled, dry and of a dirty-grayish color, has suffered for nearly six months from a watery, cadaverously smelling diarrhœa which passes involuntarily from 20 to 25 times a day. Besides, she has an enormous navel-hernia, nearly as large as a hen's egg, eats little, sleeps still less, but drinks all the time, especially cold water, greedily; the voice resembles that of a kitten. *Arsen.* 30, three drops in two ounces of water, a teaspoonful twice a day; fourteen days afterwards the child looked better, and no longer drank so much. Diarrhœa, though still passing from 10 to 15 times a day, no longer offensive. *Arsen.* as before. October 25th, 1866, her mother came to me with another child of hers afflicted with otorrhœa, and told me that Harriet had been running about lively and healthy for eighteen months (A. H. Z., 80, 15, Dr. Bojanus, in Moskau).

NOTE.—*Arsen.* and *Graph.* in alternation (continued for six months with intervals), are praised against malignant impetigo of the head upon a scrofulous bottom (also, when plica polonica exists at the same time*) (Bericht ueber die am 20. Juli, 1868, in Dortmund abgehaltene Versammlung der Homœopathen Rheinlands u. Westphalens).

## AURUM.

### GENERALITIES.

*Aurum* has many characteristic drug effects in common with *Arsen.* Thus *great difficulty of breathing during the night*, and violent *palpitation* of the heart. But as *Aurum* acts more

* Others praise here Staphisagria 1, one drop morning and evening for weeks.

decidedly upon the glandular system, it is a more useful remedy in scrofula. In the torpid form of scrofula it has been given with more success. Thus especially, *Aur. mur. natronat.* 3 trit. (according to Schweikert, of Breslau), against scrofulous glandular ulcers with torn, indented edges, and caseo-lardaceous secretion; scrofulous ulcers of the conjunctiva and cornea, but also against knotty, scirrhous glands.

Nightly pains in the bones, especially of the nasal bones, fetid smell from the nose. *Aurum*, it is true, cures ulceration of the bone, also, but more when the anamnesis allows us to infer the influence of syphilis or *Mercury*. Swelling and suppuration of the inguinal glands. Induration or swelling of the testes.

Next to *Arsenicum*, *Aurum* much resembles *Silic.* It may also be mentioned that mental depression, hence melancholic temperament, decrease of memory, rabid appetite, simultaneous affections of the gums would speak for the selection of *Aurum* (S. Dr. Bær's Beobacht. über Primärwirkg. von Gold., A. H. Z., 54, 1).

### CLINIQUE.

#### 1. (XIII.) *Ozæna.*

C., a young girl, æt. 18, suffered for several years from ozæna with caries of the nasal bones. The affected organs made so fearful a smell that doors and windows had always to be opened where the patient remained. *Aurum* 3, one dose every third day, restored her health completely.

#### 2. (XIV.) *Ozæna.*

Dr. Bær within three weeks cured a girl, æt. 13, by *Aur. met.*, who to the torment of her friends suffered for a long while from a horribly smelling nasal discharge of a purulent, viscid character, and very offensive breath. She looked almost ruddy, but somewhat "*scrofulous*" (A. H. Z., 54, 1).

#### 3. (XV.) *Chronic Inflammation of the Cornea.*

Dr. Genzke cured with *Aurum* 3, one dose every evening, a chronic keratitis in a scrofulous girl, æt. 10. The cornea of the left eye was completely opaque. All the external remedies used against the trouble had proved inefficient. The whole cornea had a marbly appearance. In the periphery of the cornea a vascular wreath, highly developed. No pain, no increased secretion of tears.

The cornea had been in this condition four months. It required eight weeks to restore its transparency (A. H. Z., 55, 10).

4. (XVI.) *Opacity of the Cornea.*

In another case *Hep. sulph.* had removed the main trouble, while *Aurum* 3, one grain every evening, restored the clearness of the cornea. Before the patient came under homœopathic treatment the power of sight was lost almost entirely; with the left eye he could not recognize anything, but merely distinguish between light and darkness; with the right eye he saw something, but could not distinguish forms and outlines of objects.

5. (XVII.) *Scrofulo-rheumatic Ophthalmia.*

That the effect of *Aurum*, in such cases, is not accidental, another cure by the same author plainly demonstrates, in which a remedial aggravation upon each single dose of the *gold* could be distinctly proven (A. H. Z., 55, 11).

Mrs. K., of D., had suffered the year previous from scrofulo-rheumatic ophthalmia which, finally, had given way to a long allopathic treatment, but left a considerable cicatrix upon the pupil of the right eye, on account of which the power of sight was much impaired. At the beginning of the new year she was affected by the same inflammation on both eyes which, in spite of the immediate curative efforts of the same physician, increased to such a degree as to enlarge the cicatrix on the right eye, and produce opacity over the whole surface of the left, so that the power of sight was entirely suspended. Conjunctiva reddened, great photophobia, burning hot tears, and violent cutting pains tortured the patient. The former physician strewed calomel into the eye, and hoped to cure the woman within the course of one year.

*Spigel.* 4, morning and evening, lessened the inflammation, afterwards *Phosph.* 30, against taking cold easily, with the result that now the inflammatory symptoms disappeared.

Now, of *Aurum* 3, which taken in doses of a whole powder daily, increased the irritability (photophobia), one grain was given every other day, which brought forth the following report: "There is, Heaven be praised, so essential an improvement that my wife is already able to read well." The complete cure (July 1st) resulted from the sole and continuous administration of *Aurum*. At the same time with it the diplopia disappeared, which was occasioned by a perpendicular cicatrix upon the cornea.

NOTE.—The experiments of Dr. v. Pratobevera do not seem to be void of interest with regard to the indications of *gold*. Aside from the boring and burning pains, accompanied by redness and swelling, even, which he felt in various parts of the body, especially in the bones of the foot, he observed that an eczematous eruption which, thus far, had not molested him any, began to discharge after itching previously, and spread considerably. The axillary glands in the neighborhood were swollen.

A dose of *Aurum* 12, taken at a later date, compelled him to give up his experiments.

## BARYTA MURIATICA.

### GENERALITIES.

*Baryt. mur.* was used for a time as an excellent antiscrofulosum, especially on Hufeland's recommendation, who advised its application in inflammatory conditions of the glands. At present its use is more limited, though *Baryt.* is equally indispensable as *Iodine*, and in its place equally efficacious. It is true the indications regarding its application cannot be given so definitely. Its physiological effects upon the glandular system were principally observed in the tonsils and axillary glands. As a therapeutic effect it was observed that, during its administration, scrofulous and other glandular swellings decreased, and inflamed glands became more painful.

Of the several preparations, *Baryt. mur.* seems to act more energetically than *Baryt. acet.*, and the latter less than *Baryt. carb.* (Dr. Reil in N. Z. f. h. Kl., 1, 10).

While *gold* corresponds to the torpid forms of scrofula, *Baryt.* is indicated in all forms of scrofulosis florida (glandular indurations and swellings) (Altschul). Also in hypertrophy of the thyroid gland (struma), induration of the mamma; in tumor albus (Lisfranc), a specific in existing predisposition to angina.* Among the characteristic drug effects, *Baryt.* has even swelling of the testes in common with *Aurum.*

According to the valuable experiences of Dr. Altmueller, of Cassel, the sphere of action of *Baryt. mur.* is principally the lymphatic and glandular system, and the tissues standing upon the same step of organization with the former. *Its curative effects are confirmed only in scrofulous diseases, scrofulous ophthalmia, scrofulous cutaneous eruptions and diarrhœa* resulting therefrom, as well as in *pulmonary blennorrhœa.*

Dr. Altmueller, in our opinion, is the first who has pointed here to the connection of scrofula with certain affections of the mucosa of the respiratory organs. Most surely, however, there exists such a connection. The proof of it must be of the greatest importance to therapeutics. It is, no doubt, more generally known that, among the diseases of the upper portion of the organs of respiration, *i. e.*, of the larynx; croup frequently enough coincides with the most developed habitus scrofulosus. For this reason the specific beneficial influence of the genuine antiscrofulosa, *Hepar.*, *Calc.*, *Spong.*, *Iod.*, and *Brom.* This connection, marked out by Altmueller, becomes still more evident, if one reminds himself of the cases so frequent in practice, from which, after spontaneous or non-spontaneous disappearance of a scrofulous cutaneous eruption, an obstinate cough (bronchitis), and even pneumonia, with copious expectoration, result. But we have, also, frequently enough opportunity of observing that scrofulous diarrhœa appears as a substitute. That the diarrhœa is a scrofulous one, is plain from the fact that the antiscrofulosum, *Calc. carb.*, corresponds to it in the most effective manner.

"The application of *Baryta mur.*," Altmueller further says, "I have found most powerful in the following fluid form: One

* Dr. Zwingenberg (Brandenburg) recommends against scrofulous hypertrophy of the tonsils: Liquor. baryt. mur. one drop in one-half a cupful of lukewarm water, as a gargarisma, from two to three times a day, with intermissions, used for weeks.

scruple (1, 2) of the third trit. in four tablespoonfuls of distilled water. Of this a child one year of age was given a tablespoonful every three hours; and in this way the quantity of doses was increased or decreased, according to age and individuality.*

CLINIQUE.

### 1. (XVIII.) *Atrophia. Abdominal Scrofula.*

The son of Mr. A., a child two years of age, suffered from atrophia. The whole neck, covered with indurated glands of egg-size; the abdomen much distended and hard; the seventh and eighth dorsal vertebræ grown out into a hump; from both ears discharge of offensive pus; tongue coated; stool produced by enemata only; the fæces, small in quantity, as hard as a stone, and white of color; the urine yellowish, very offensive; the feet swollen. Such was the pathological picture when I was called, after an unsuccessful allopathic treatment of many (years ?†) months. I gave twenty grains of the third trit. of *Baryt. mur.* in four tablespoonfuls of distilled water, a teaspoonful three times a day. The vegetable diet, consisting of mucilaginous food, the animal diet of milk only. To counteract the progress in the dislocation of the vertebræ, the child was laid upon a sand-pillow one hand in width and one foot long, corresponding to the dislocated part. An injection of oil and water was given every day. In the course of fourteen days the child improved from day to day and became more lively; appetite returned, especially for milk; the urine changed for the better. Three months afterwards all troubles had subsided; no trace is left of the dislocation of the vertebræ, and the boy is now well and healthy. He received no other remedy but *Baryt. mur.*, and took twelve doses, such as mentioned, during the whole treatment.

---

* Dr. A. triturated four grains of baryt. mur. with ninety-six grains of sach. lact., and prepared from this the second, and from this again the third trit.

† Dr. A. seems to have forgotten that the child was only two years old.

### 2. (XIX.) *Atrophia.*

E. K., æt. 1½, was covered with ulcers over the whole body; the whole head with thick, offensive crusts; abscesses behind the ears, which discharged an offensive pus; fetid discharge from the ears like rotten cheese; both eyelids swollen; the bulbs of the eye very much inflamed; photophobia, so that the child always lay upon its face; abdomen considerably swollen; thin, watery, very offensive stools; both feet very much swollen.

Sixteen grains of *Baryt. mur.*, third trit., in three tablespoonfuls of distilled water, a teaspoonful three times a day, improved before the exhaustion of the solution to such a degree as to completely restore health within six months; and now, a year from the time, a healthy and fleshy girl has developed from this complete picture of misery, for whom the parents had frequently wished liberation from her sufferings by death. During the treatment, the dose was increased two grains from time to time.

### 3. (XX.) *Ophthalmia Scrofulosa.*

The daughter of shoemaker G., æt. 6, was afflicted with scrofulous ophthalmia, and was treated for a whole year by the allopathic physician Dr. Stilling. After Dr. S. had dismissed her as incurable, I undertook the treatment of the child, her condition being then as follows: Total opacity of the cornea; the sclerotica inflamed and loosened in its tissue; entire blindness; both nasal openings sore and inflamed. She received 20 grains of *Baryt. mur.*, in four tablespoonfuls of distilled water, half a tablespoonful three times a day. After a treatment of three weeks the ophthalmia disappeared, and four months afterwards the child's eyes were entirely clear, and her power of sight complete.

## BROMIUM.

### GENERALITIES.

By its continued use enlargement of glandular organs and swellings of the lymphatics were observed to disappear; but from its similarity to *Iodium*, its similar physiological action and therapeutic usefulness were inferred. Especially Glower frequently applied *Kal. brom.*, successfully in scrofula and chronic diseases of the glands (Dr. Reil in N. Z. f. h. Kl., 2, 9).

*The celebrated springs of Kreuznach (Elizabeth-spring) owe their antiscrofulous action, aside from* Iod., *to their contents of* Bromium.

*Brom.* has been warmly recommended by Gauwerky against obstinate scrofulous affections, and by Hofrichter, against suppuration of the glands.

Among its characteristic, pathogenetic effects are: Flow of tears; burning in the mouth and œsophagus; cough and paroxysms of suffocation; impeded respiration and gasping for air; stitches in the lungs while breathing; glandular affections. Its action upon the organs of respiration, and among the glandular organs, upon the thyroid gland and testicles, is remarkable.

Succor has been obtained in membranous croup from the *vapors* of *Brom.*, when *Iod.* had failed.* Upon the whole, the cures of scrofulous affections effected by *Bromine* may be principally divided into such as pertain either to *glandular diseases* or *croup.*

As regards the dose, Dr. Kaesemann remarks that *Brom.* would prove itself most efficacious, probably, in the lower dilutions. He bases his opinion upon a passage of the H. M. M. of Noack and Trinks which reads as follows: "If the volatility of a remedy constitutes a reason for its application in the lower grades of dilution and more frequent repetition; this rule will be worth observing with regard to the administration of *Bromine.*"

### CLINIQUE.

#### 1. (XXI.) *Cure of Croup.*

K. W., æt. 1½, feeble, descending from rhachitic parents, and living upon unhealthy food, pot-bellied and of scrofulo-

* Pathological anatomy teaches us that swelling and induration of the mesenterial glands, inflammation of the larynx and air-passages with exudations of a plastic lymph (inflammation and hypertrophy of the heart), result from toxical doses of Bromine.

rhachitic habitus. About eight days ago she had an intense coryza which *suddenly disappeared previous to her sickness.* For a few days past the child has suffered from hoarseness which has so increased since evening that at 9 P.M. entire aphonia has set in; besides, very laborious, long-drawn inspirations, at times resembling snoring;—according to report previously mucous rattling to such a degree, as to make one fear suffocation. Cough is absent; temperature of the skin but little raised; no thirst; she does not wish to eat anything; during the day she has still eaten and played.

*Brom.* 0, 3, six drops in twelve teaspoonfuls of water, a teaspoonful from one-quarter to one-half hour. Better; she has already left her bed for several hours. After *Bromium relief had set in at once;* cough and expectoration had appeared, something that recurred several times through the night.

One dose of the above prescription every hour, 9 P.M., I was told that her condition had grown worse again, considerably; return of aphonia with mucous rattling on respiration, so much so, that suffocation was feared; the skin covered with cold sweat.

*Brom.* 0, 3, nine drops from one-quarter to one-half hour.

Had left her bed next day, though she had perspired much during the night. Cough, the evening previous barking and laborious, to-day more sonorous, easy, moist and more frequent, seldom during the night, though accompanied by much rattling and difficulty of breathing. The same prescription.

The child, although poorly cared for, recovered under the continued use of *Brom.* within a few days.

It was discontinued, however, when slight coughing up of blood and nose-bleed set in. Dr. Kæsemann considers the latter symptoms to be the effects of *Bromium;* from this it is self-evident, no doubt, that the dose might be a smaller one, and, indeed, very brilliant results have been obtained since with higher dilutions given at long intervals (S. the next cure, but also No. 8*). Moreover, in another cure of genuine croup (by Kali bichr.), blood and bloody mucus were coughed up at the termination of the disease.

---

* Heilungen von Croup, Croupine, Asthma, &c., mit Brom. von Dr. Kæsemann in Lich. (A H. Z., 48, 24).

### 2. (XXII.) *Cure of Croup.*

Of the many cases of croup cured by Dr. Kirsch, of Wiesbaden, we will report but the following (A. H. Z., 47, 18):

Dec. 7th, 1853. Mrs. M. came to Dr. K., requesting him to give her a remedy against an attack of croup in her niece, æt. 5, who had been treated for three days already, by two allopathic physicians, with emetics. Since the disease showed no amelioration, they had agreed to perform the operation of tracheotomy in the evening.

Aconit. $\frac{000}{\times}$, and Brom. $\frac{000}{\times}$, each powder to be dissolved in a separate tumbler, containing three tablespoonfuls of water. Of these solutions a teaspoonful every twenty minutes alternately.

Three hours afterwards (at 6 P.M.) K. was told that the physicians had come between 5 and 6 P.M.; but as they had been at the eve of taking out their instruments, had heard the changed sound of the cough, looked at each other in surprise, and remarked: "The operation is not required any more, but continue with the powders (pointing to the Sulphate of copper prescribed by them), and when they are all taken, send for another supply forthwith." K. was informed that after taking the first, and especially the second remedy, a visible relief, steadily progressing, had set in; that the child, before cold and blue, with the terrible tight and barking cough, had broken out in a warm sweat, and that the cough soon had become changed, *i. e.*, got looser and soluble.

Seventy-two hours afterwards the same remedies, now dissolved in four tablespoonfuls of water, were given at longer intervals, until a complete recovery set in, accompanied by a general sweat and loose expectoration.

At the close Dr. Kirsch combats Dr. Lutze's assertion that a child, homœopathically treated for croup, would never have a return of it. The return, Dr. K. says, was prevented only after the scrofulous affection, which was at the bottom of it, was entirely removed by the proper remedies (and, probably by means of a more correct diet)!

### 3. (XXIII.) *Cures of Croup.*

The A. H. Z. (48, 22, and 24, and 49, 16), contains interesting cures by *Brom.*, especially in croup and affections related to it. *Loc. cit.*, Dr. Kæsemann designates *Brom.* as, probably, the grandest remedy in croup. Dr. Kirsch, of Wiesbaden, has had similar experiences, which he has published in A. H. Z., 46, and 47, 141, &c.

### 4. (XXIV.) *Cure of Croup.*

In a desperate case of croup in a feeble, scrofulous girl, æt. 5, *Spong.*, *Hep.*, and *Brom.* 30, were unable to arrest the increase of the disease. But upon the use of *Brom.* $1^x$, six drops to two ounces (60, 0) of water, a teaspoonful from one-half to two hours, improvement set in slowly.

A highly interesting case was cured only after *Phos.* 1 and *Brom.* 2 had been given (A. H. Z., 53, 14, Theuerkauf.).

### 5. (XXV.) *Cure of Croup.*

In the A. H. Z., 54, 2, a cure of a case of intense torpid croup is communicated by Dr. Elb, in which *Brom.* 3 (two drops every hour) likewise averted the danger to life* (after *Acon.* 2 and *Iod.* 3 had been given in vain). But upon returning aggravation he was compelled to give *Brom.* in alternation with *Hep. s.* 2 (gr. ij). "With the disappearance of the croup, coryza had appeared." When refuge was taken with *Brom.* the first time, Dr. Elb found the boy, æt. 2½, icy cold, the breathing short, superficial, and violently sawing; the head bent back, the face pale and bloated, the lips blue, the pulse very weak and rapid; total aphonia; the eyes set; *cough had been absent almost totally for two hours.* The remark interponed here by Dr. Elb is of interest: "During a practice of nineteen years it was the first time that *Iod.* failed to do its service in such a case, apparently so suitable for it."

### 6. (XXVI.) *Cure of Croup.*

In L'Art. Méd., Jan., 1858, cure of a violent case of croup by *Brom.*; Dr. Milcent.

---

* Dr. Elb calls croup "torpid" on account of the slow development and long duration of the cough, comparatively rare; the degree of dyspnœa, slight, upon the whole, and absence of synochal fever; though a considerable quantity of exudation was present.

The child was seven years old, had a rough cough, violent fever, and pain in the throat. Two days afterwards the voice became hoarse, the cough more dry, respiration more difficult; a rough, dry whistling, seated in the larynx, accompanied every breath of air; the fever increased; delirium; paroxysms of suffocation; the child lay on its back with a pale and somewhat livid face; totally aphonous; breathing frequent and short; pulse 160; now restless, now comatose; the short, dry cough threatened to suffocate it; skin burning hot; the pseudo-membranous exudations confined to the larynx; while coughing the child vomited up, now and then, a serous liquid, in which shreds of the pseudo-membranes were observed.

*Brom.* 4, gtt. 4, in 125, 0 of water, every two hours, effected at least an arrest of the progress of the trouble for two days; indeed, the paroxysms of suffocation had become less frequent, and the fever less. Upon renewed hourly doses of the remedy (*Brom.* 4, gtt. 10, in 240, 0 of water), the improvement was surprising, and ended with complete recovery; the hoarseness lasted longest.

## BROMINE IN SCROFULOUS GLANDULAR AFFECTIONS.

### 7. (XXVII.) *Affection of the Mesenterial Glands.*

Dr. Hilberger, of Trieste, communicates, in his "Klinischen Beobachtungen" (Z. f. h. Kl., 2, 15), a very interesting case of "scrofulous infiltrations of the mesenterial glands and chronic pneumonia," in which *Brom.* 6 effected the resorption of the mesenterial glands after *Arsen.* 6, in alternation with *Carb. veg.* 6, had removed the existing œdematous swelling and intense dyspnœa, in short, the pneumonic portion of the disease, which did not point by any means to a spontaneous improvement, not to say recovery. It is probable that *Carb. veget.* also had influence upon the resorption within the glands.

"Of late Hofrichter says, I have sufficiently convinced myself of the extraordinary and sure effect of *Brom.* in scrofulous affections, *i. e.*, in inveterate indurated and already partly suppurating glandular swellings. I began my experiments with the 15th dilution, descended, however, to the 6th, and believe that the latter is to be preferred to the former, since by its aid glandular swellings and indurations soften more rapidly without in any way affecting the rest of the organism."

8. (XXVIII.) *Scrofulous Affections of the Cervical Glands.*

H. H., pupil of the Polytechnic Institute, æt. 20, has suffered four years from swollen suppurating cervical glands on the right side. There is, likewise, a hard painful gland of the size of a fist, studded with several cicatrices, still suppurating, in the right axilla, which hinders him especially in drawing, and threatens to compel him from continuing his studies. The neighboring glands feel like large peas, and some still larger; he has to carry the arm in a sling, to keep the upper arm at a distance from the chest; cold lodging; poor food.

Jan. 15th, 1852. *Sulphur* 60, four doses; every second day one powder. A month afterwards pain less; swelling somewhat smaller.

Feb. 17th. *Silic.* 30 in the same manner. First the glandular swelling seemed to increase in size, discharged a good deal of pus, but finally the openings seemed to have closed up.

March 26th. *Calc. carb.* 30. Upon its use for two months the glandular swelling decreased, broke open again a few times, and healed again, but finally a standstill took place, and *Calcar.* did not seem to exert any subsequent effect.

Aug. 1st. *Brom.* 15. Fourteen days afterwards the axillary glands became painful, blisters formed upon its surface, which broke and developed into suppurating ulcers; yet, in proportion to the suppuration the swelling decreased. His general health improved remarkably, and his face assumed a healthy complexion.

*Brom.* was continued for a whole year, whereupon the enlargement of the cervical and axillary glands had been resorbed, and the best health followed.

9. (XXIX.) *Scrofulous Glandular Affection.*

A youth, æt. 17, suffered from his childhood from swollen cervical glands. When he came to Dr. N. he could wear no neckcloth; the left submaxillary gland was twice as large as a walnut, and hung down on the neck like a bag; on the right side the glands were swollen to the size of hazelnuts. They were, however, not painful, and not sensitive upon touch, though several parts thereof during the treatment became red and painful, and made us suspect suppuration, but the the process always ended with resorption.

He was treated for nine months with *Brom.* 6, one powder every forty-eight hours, and the swellings disappeared completely.

What important relations exist between the curative effects of *Brom.* and the scrofula-dyscrasia, that just the presence of the latter, if we are undecided among several remedies, decides for *Brom.*, evidently seems to follow from the following clinical observations of the same author.

### 10. (XXX.) *Chronic Swelling of the Tonsils.*

A boy, æt. 8, after preceding chronic inflammation of both eyes, suffered from such extensive opacities of the cornea as to compel him to roll the eyes in a horrible manner, in order to distinguish the road before him; the lids swollen and knotty to the touch; purulent discharge of the swollen conjunctiva palpebrarum; besides, the child was deaf in consequence of the disease. Inspection of the throat showed very large tonsils; otorrhœa had been present previously. The whole face bloated; the nose thick; continuous and offensive coryza; lips swollen; most of the teeth carious, and the submaxillary glands as large as walnuts, but painless. Yet notwithstanding all this *Brom.* 6, one powder every forty-eight hours, made such an improvement as to enable his parents to send him to the country. The glandular swellings, as well as the deafness, had disappeared with the decrease of the tonsilar enlargement. Even the opacities of the cornea were removed so far that the darkest portion only looked opaque; the lids returned to their normal form; the chronic inflammation of the conjunctiva, and thus its swollen condition, even, disappeared, as well as the discharge from the nose, in consequence of which the swelling of nose and lips went down naturally.

NOTE.—Dr. Kallenbach has often prescribed *Brom.* or *Kal. brom.* 6 in scrofulous affections, but cannot maintain that it has done any more than the well-known remedies, *Sulph.*,

*Calc.*, *Iod.*, *Con.*, when closely corresponding to the individual case. He deems it specific, however, in chronic ovaritis, such as may be found in young women who have had no children. (A. H. Z., 50, 1.)

### 11. (XXXI.) *Affection of the Submaxillary Glands.*

Theuerkauf fully confirms the efficacy of *Brom.* in scrofulous affections, especially in stone-hard swellings of the glands, such as are wont to appear on the lower jaw and neck of scrofulous subjects.

A poor scrofulous girl, æt. 14, with blonde hair and rosy cheeks, who had suffered for a long time from a hard swelling of the submaxillary glands, and taken against it various homœopathic remedies with but little result, received *Brom.* 30, one dose every fourth day. The remedy having been continued for some time, she may now be discharged as cured. When *Brom.* 30 was given the left submaxillary gland had reached the size of a small hen's-egg, was hard, painless upon touch, and the neighboring glands were affected more or less in the same manner.

### 12. (XXXII.) *Affection of a Submaxillary Gland.*

A scrofulous youth, æt. 16, for several years had a hard, painless, and swollen gland, as large as half a hen's egg, at the right side of the lower jaw. Allopathic remedies had been fruitless.

He took *Brom.* 30 four times (as above). This caused a reduction of the gland to the size of a hazelnut; and, when Theuerkauf made inquiries, afterwards, this rest of the trouble even had disappeared* (A. H. Z., 53, 22).

## CALCAREA CARBONICA.

### GENERALITIES.

Water that contains the salts of lime in excess (and deposits drop-stone in its course) is accused by some of produc-

* Dr. Gerson saw good results from Merc. bijodat., if the tuberous, scrofulo-glandular swellings were accompanied by intense redness of the skin, but very little pain (A. H. Z., 54, 5).

ing scrofula. Thus it is said that the inhabitants of Rheims owe the large number of persons affected by scrofula among their population to this circumstance. Does there exist a greater triumph to Hahnemann's discovery? The Hahnemannian school, if it were to do without the salts of lime, would not wish to treat scrofula. *Calc. carb.* performs wonders in scrofulous ophthalmia; like *Sulph.*, it removes scrofulous pot-bellies, if I may be allowed to use this expression; like *Phos.*, it cures scrofulous diarrhœa, &c.

It acts, to express it in general terms, directly upon the ganglionic system and the organs under its control, but especially upon the skin and intestinal mucosa.*

*Calcarea*, another author says, has but few specific relations to single organs, but has bearings of a decided and well-marked character upon definite tissues and organic systems, and to the whole process of formation and reformation—to the life of the blood.

Of the tissues and organic systems upon which *Calc.* shows a well-defined action, the *glandular* system, *osseous tissue*, and *mucous membranes* must be marked out especially.

Thus *Calcar.* principally suits in those diseases and individualities in whom the process of formation and reformation is exposed to disturbances—the age of childhood, the female sex, the lymphatic and leucæmic constitutions; moreover, in the process of dentition, in scrofulosis, rhachitis, chlorosis, arthritis, and lithiasis (N. Z. f. h. Kl.).

Dr. Reil's general remarks upon this remedy finally agree with this. In therapeutics, he resumes, the preparations of lime (*Calc. acet.*, *carb. caustic.*, *phosphor.*, *muriat.*, and *sulphurata; Hep. sulph. calc.*) have played a great part as remedies for the glands, antidyscratica, antiscrofulosa, and antilymphatica; pharmacodynamists, such as Vogt, Richter, and Greiner, ascribe to it the direct power of producing a specific internal change in vegetation; a specific influence upon the

* "The carbonate of lime predominates in the non-vertebrate animals with pale-looking ganglia, the phosphate appearing at the same time in the vertebrates. Phosphate of lime genetically is the contrarium to the medulla nervea. A rapid waste of nerve force immediately occasions, hence an equally rapid production of earths, of which the carbonate of lime again corresponds to the ganglionic system, the phosphate to the cerebro-spinal."

nervous system of the entire lymphatic and glandular system (especially upon the mesenterial glands).

In view of the characteristic pathogenetic effects of *Calc. carb.*, such as glandular swellings, ophthalmia scrofulosa (opacity of the cornea), otorrhœa; discharge of an offensive fluid from the nose; distension of the abdomen; constipation (but also diarrhœa), the remedy has been tried and found efficacious in the various manifestations of scrofulosis:

1. In crusta lactea, acne, facial eczema, impetigo, pemphigus, and onychia, especially when acidity of the stomach is present.
2. In scrofulous degeneration of the mesenterial, thyroid (struma), and cervical glands.
3. In chronic headaches of scrofulous persons.
4. In ophthalmia scrofulosa.
5. In otorrhœa purulenta scrofulosa.
6. In ozæna scrofulosa with loss of smell, as well as against the formation of polypi.
7. In dyspepsia, accompanied by water-brash and eructations with the taste of the food taken.
8. In habitual diarrhœa, sour-smelling diarrhœa of children; ascarides.
9. In incipient rhachitis (walking of children at a late date), difficult dentition of infants, slowly-closing fontanels.

*Caustic.* and *Lycopod.* much resemble *Calcar. carb.*

*Caustic.* is indicated also in strumatous swellings, in pustular eruptions, moist eczema, scrofulous otorrhœa; (nervous) dyspepsia; panaritium; ophth. scrof. of a chronic character, with spots upon the cornea; but it is hardly possible to confound them, if we consider that *Caustic.* (like *Rhus*) corresponds more to the rheumatic than scrofulous diathesis.

At the head of the *Caustic.* symptoms stand arthritic and rheumatic tearing in the limbs; contractions of the limbs, with paralysis; paralysis after apoplexy; pain as from luxation in the hip-joint, &c.

It is more difficult to draw a line between *Calcar.* and *Lycopod.*, since both complement and not oppose each other in their action. *Lycop.* resembles *Sulphur*, but the fact that *Calcar. carb.* does excellent service in suppressed hæmorrhoids and their evil consequences—(Richter recommends here injections of lime-water)—hence is an anti-hæmorrhoidale—shows how closely related in their action *Calc.* and *Sulph.* are. In absence of other points of support, we may say that the diseases cured by *Lycopod.* are more frequently associated with disturbances of the liver than is the case with *Calcar.* Hence, the yellowish (greenish) color of the secretions (yellowish complexion, yellowish tongue, yellowish sputa), &c.

*Lycopod.* suits (probably for this reason) oftener in diseases of grown persons; *Silic.*, *Graph.*, and *Arsen.* resemble *Lycopod.* more than *Calcar.*

*Calcarea* is indicated in many cases before *Lycopod.*, in the first stage, so to say, when an opposite condition has not followed, as yet, upon exaltation. In connection therewith *Lycopodium* more than *Calcar.* has "*obstruction*" in a more extended sense of the word.

When *Lycopod.* exceptionally cures diarrhœa (*Sulph.* exceptionally does the same), it has been, then, so to say, a secondary diarrhœa, a sequela to preceding constipation. *Calcar.*, however, is a specific remedy in innumerable cases of diarrhœa of teething, scrofulous infants, which, probably, may constitute reflex-phenomena, yet do not deserve the name secondary.

In short, *Calcarea carbonica* is a more sovereign remedy against scrofula than *Lycopod.* Besides *Silic.* and *Phosph.*, it is the *antiscrofulosum par excellence.*

## CLINIQUE.

### 1. (XXXIII.)

A boy, æt. 6, on account of the continuous use of purgatives for expelling worms, fell a victim to scrofulous atrophia, which resisted all homœopathic remedies applied, even *Calc. carb.* 12, until upon giving the 6th potency of the same remedy, prepared by a thousand arm-strokes,* a rapid and complete cure was effected, and even the glandular swellings and the hard abdomen entirely disappeared.

---

* Memorabilien aus der Praxis von Dr. Wahle in Rom. S.S., 17–50. The author believes that powerful and long-continued shaking calls forth a greater medicinal efficacy, and that the whole mystery of Jehnichen's high potencies mainly rests upon this manœuvre.

### 2. (XXXIV.) *Otorrhœa.*

Dr. Rentsch, of Potsdam, reports instructive cases of catarrh of the meat. audit. ext. in originally scrofulous individuals by *Calc. carb.* They are instructive for the reason that they testify to the possibility of a lull in scrofulosis, lasting for years, as well as show that the sudden disappearance of habitual otorrhœa has bad consequences; that, moreover, if such a morbid drying up takes place, the lymphatics swell, and that the scrofulous materia peccans moves thither, as it were.*

In one case, *Ferr. metal.* 1, ten grains morning and evening had to be given besides *Calc. carb.*, the patient being a chlorotic girl, eleven years of age.

### 3. (XXXV.) *Scrofulous Inflammation of the Knee.*

Dr. Kallenbach, of Cleve, describes the *Calcarea*—affections of the knee-joint,† and says that they attack mostly scrofulous individuals. Slight digestive disturbances, loss of appetite, irregularity in the stools are present. The pains are bearable (in contradistinction to the *Baryta*-affections of the knee-joint), pressing and stinging, intermitting at night and when at rest, worse in going up and down stairs (flexion).

Very often the trouble aggravates at the time of the full moon. Swelling, if present at all, at the inner and lower side. The painful spot at the inner side of the patella.

In his "Klinischen Beobachtungen," Dr. Hilberger, of Trieste, compares *Calc. carb.* with *Conium*, and says: "While the curative power of *Con.* confines itself to the softening of the induration, the effect of *Calc.* is more marked. It corresponds upon the whole to the scrofula-dyscrasia. That this, without having manifested itself in childhood, may become the cause of many diseases, frequently in an advanced age, every practitioner will have convinced himself."

Its special relation to glandular affections is equally evident, and fully justifies its application (Z. f. h. Kl., 3, 14).

---

* Beitraege zur Erkenntniss und Behandlung einiger Ohren Krankheiten v. Dr. Rentsch XXXVI, 1, 6.

† 52, S. 51.

But that *Calc. carb.* has a more extended sphere than the glands, and especially corresponds to the affections of the mucous membranes, the organs of sense and their auxiliary apparatuses, the cures of polypi of the mucous membranes by *Calc. carb.* prove among others.

4. (XXXVI.) *Cure of a Polypus.*

Goullon, Sr., reports an interesting case of nasal polypus which had enlarged so much as seemingly to render an operation necessary. Twelve doses of *Calc. carb.* 30, one dose a day; afterwards eight doses of the 18th dil. and lastly of the 9th dil. taken in the same manner, effected so rapid a reduction and withering of the polypus that fourteen days after taking the second medicine but a fold of the mucosa remained. The cure still continued two years afterwards (A. H. Z., 45, 5).

5. (XXXVII.) *Cure of a Polypus.*

In the N. Z. f. h. Kl., 3, 3, we find the cure of a polypus by *Calc. carb.* 9.

A woman, æt. 54, who had suffered from eight to nine years from continual hoarseness, received *Calc. carb.* 9, a dose every fourth day. After about eight days' use of this remedy, cough set in which was dry, whistling, and spasmodic, and a few days afterwards occasioned the expectoration of firm, fleshy pieces from the size of a hemp-seed to that of a pea which, on closer examination, showed themselves to be polypous masses, and thus gave information of the cause of the hoarseness of many years' standing. After from ten to twelve such pieces had been coughed up, the cough ceased, and nothing of a similar kind reappeared, notwithstanding the longer continued use of *Calc. carb.* Though Dr. Buerkner who made this observation, did not conceal the fact that the hoarseness itself continued unchanged, he yet is right, no doubt, in ascribing to *Calc. carb.* a direct influence upon the life of the polypus.

6. (XXXVIII.) *Ophthalmia Scrofulosa.*

J. L., æt. 6, of a well-marked scrofulous habitus, pale, bloated face, very much distended abdomen, and emaciated extremities, has suffered for two years from scrofulous ophthalmia which, thus far, has been combated with all sorts of remedies, but not cured.

Eyelids much swollen and inflamed, the cornea of the right eye, just in the centre opposite the pupil, shows a pearly-gray, lymphatic turbidity of considerable extent, non-transparent in its centre, and as large as a lentil. Conjunct. palpebr. loosened, conjunct. bulbi much injected. Excessive photophobia; burning pain in the eye, if she looks toward the window, with a stream of tears running over the cheeks simultaneously.

After the necessary regulation of diet, *Calcar. carb.* 3 was prescribed in daily alternation with *Sulphur* 3, and the result was surprising, indeed. Within ten days the inflammation proper, with its concomitant symptoms, was removed almost entirely, and the spot on the cornea grew smaller, so as to disappear entirely within the course of four weeks. (Pract. Mittheil. v. Dr. Perutz, A. H. Z., 54, 6.)

### 7. (XXXIX.) *Impetigo.*

Dr. Cramoisy treated a case of impet. figurata.* The patient, æt. 20, was of lymphatic temperament; when a child, had had tinea and a scrofulous ulcer upon the thigh. The eruption, slightly itching, spread from the left cheek over to the right, the chin, and the entire face, almost. *Calc. carb.* 6, two drops in 250, 0 of water, a teaspoonful three times a day, gave the first impulse to a cure. Afterwards, however, *Hep.*, *Graphit.*, and, lastly, *Calcar.* and *Sulphur* in alternation, were given (Journal de la Soc. Gallic. de Méd. Hom., 15 Mai, 1857).

### 8. (XL.) *Cures of Cysts.*

In L'art. Médical, October and December, 1866, we find some very instructive cures with *Calc. carb.* (Dr. Bourgeois), the names of which we will mention merely, since the persons cured are not expressly mentioned as having been scrofulous. He cured:

Three cysts at the knee.

---

* First described by Willan. Impetig. fig. possesses the characteristic of assuming the form of the part upon which it takes its seat.

One cyst on the finger.
One cyst at the metacarpal joint.
Two cysts at the eyelid.
One cyst on the breast.
Lipomata.
Three times warts on the face and hands.

### 9. (XLI.) *Cure of Struma.*

M. D., æt. 10, of rosy complexion and delicate musculature, suffers from rheumatism and diarrhœa. Aversion to meat.

Was affected in his seventh year by goitre, against which *Iodine* preparations and *Spongia* were given in vain; on the contrary, the swelling increased all the time. No treatment for the past six months. The tumor is located to the left, anteriorly, as large as a pigeon's egg, soft, doughy, painless, movable, and pervaded by blue veins.

May 16th. *Calc. carb.*, 15 centigrammes of the third trit. every day for ten days.

A month later the appetite had improved, but the humor was not changed essentially.

*Calc. carb.* 6, six drops in 200, 0 of water; a teaspoonful morning and evening.

July 10th. Remarkable improvement; struma decreased in circumference, and otorrhœa of one year's standing disappeared. *Calc. carb.* 3.

The struma has grown decidedly smaller during September, and toward the end of the year is completely cured. (A. H. Z., 94, 6.)

### 10. (XLII.) *Cure of Struma.*

Lucie J., æt. 17, of delicate, scrofulous constitution, formerly suffering from swollen submaxillary glands, which had suppurated three times, from her 15th year on; menstruated from every six weeks to two months.

Oct. 28th, 1869, a strumatous swelling, that had made its appearance at the time of puberty, is as large as a hen's egg. Both lobes are affected. The swelling is soft and painless. At the time of menstruation patient notices an increase of the tumor, especially if the flow is scanty; then difficulty of breathing sets in also, compelling her repeatedly to jump up at night.

*Calc. carb.* 3, trit. 0, 12 centigrammes for twelve days; a dose every evening.

Three weeks afterwards, menstruation, more copious, appears at the 26th day. The struma has not increased any during the menses. No difficulty of respiration.

The same prescription.

Dec. 20th. Considerable improvement of the struma, which appears softer, less tense, and prominent. Menses after four weeks.

*Calc. carb.* 6, six drops in 200, 0 of water, two tablespoonfuls every day. At the end of January the swelling was unmistakably decreasing in size.

*Calc. carb.* 30.

During the course of March there is but a single spot at the neck which transgresses the normal level; nothing is seen, however, if one is not looking at it intently.

Dr. Bourgeois's method, in a long-continuing treatment to run over the entire scala of the Hahnemannian posology, is not at all unessential.

### 11. (XLIII.) *Cure of Struma.*

Miss K., æt. 19, affected with a considerable swelling of the thyroid gland, the increase of which she notices since a few days, and the origin of which she is not able to account for, wished to be freed from it. Difficult respiration, on lying on the back during sleep, is the only complaint made.

*Brom.* 0, 3, one drop in a tablespoonful of water, three times a day. No change within ten days.

*Calc. carb.* 0, 3, morning and evening, as much as will lay upon the point of a pocket-knife.

Eight days afterwards noticeable decrease of the swelling. Complete cure after three weeks more.

Dr. A. Starke, of Nagy Károlyi, remarks, upon this case, that Miss K. previously had been treated allopathically for one year, yet, without noticing the smallest change in her condition (*i. e.*, the smallest change for the better); for the famous Iodine-coryza appeared frequently, since she had been advised continually to apply Iod. tincture and a salve of Iodide of Potass.

### 12. (XLIV.) *Melitagra.*

Thin, yellowish, crusty eruption (melitagra of Alibert) at the right temple in a stout girl, æt. 29, who still showed the residues of scrofula, cured by *Calc. carb.* 4, one drop every other day; afterwards *Calc. carb.* 30, two globules, and *Calc. carb.* 1 gtt. j (A. H. Z., 21, 13, Dr. Frank, of Osterode).

### 13. (XLV.) *Blepharoblennorrhœa Scrofulosa,*

In a scrofulous girl, 10 years old, which had existed for several years, and had frequently been treated externally without any success, was completely cured within four weeks by *Calc. carb.* 2, and *Sulphur.* 1 (Bd. XXI, 13. Reported in the catalogue of patients received in the hom. department of the Elizabeth Hospital of Berlin, from August 20th to November 26th, 1841).

### 14. (XLVI.) *Fibrous Polypus.*

Dr. Gross, of Regensburg: Fibrous polypus cured by *Calc. carb.* $4^x$ trit., dissolved in diluted alcohol, two drops a day.

The patient, the son of a peasant, æt. 12, was of lymphatic constitution, and frequently disposed to scrofulous affections; cough, hoarseness, difficulty of swallowing, and coryza were the beginning of the trouble (A. H. Z., 57, 12).

### 15. (XLVII.) *Spondylarthrocace.*

In the last number of Vol. 73, of the A. H. Z., we find a very good report of a cure by *Calc. carb.* by Anton Starke, practical physician of Pesth, in which all the advantages and peculiar medicinal virtues of the remedy come to view.

Before the appearance of the trouble, patient was tormented by cough and backache. Fever and weakness compelled her, finally, to stay in bed continually. For two months she had been treated allopathically without any success. Lately she suffered violent pains of a boring character in the region of the last cervical and first thoracic vertebræ. She also felt drawing pain in both shoulder-blades and along the spinal column. She could not hold up her head without support from one hand or the other.

Status præsens: H. B., æt. 16, of middle size, considerably emaciated. Cheeks reddened. Thorax flat. Notwithstanding the suspicious short cough, no demonstrable abnormity of the lungs or heart. Sounds of liver and spleen also normal. Abdomen distended but not painful. Secretion of urine somewhat retarded; bowels somewhat constipated. Boring pain in the last cervical and first thoracic vertebræ. Arms feel as if they were asleep, now and then, and heaviness of the head. The whole day she remains in a semi-recumbent position. Appetite keener than ever. Thirst increased. Menstruation not set in for two months.

Processus spinosi of the seventh cervical and first three thoracic vertebræ are very much protuberant and, upon touch, show themselves to be larger in size. Upon pressure, pain increases. During the hours of the morning, fever that increases in the evening. Palms of the hands hot. The skin dry, at the same time. Pulse 104. Depressed in mind.

Diagnosis: Spondylarthrocace.

The symptoms of *Calc. carb.* correspond mostly to the above:

1. Melancholia and mental depression.
576. Ravenous appetite.
801. Hard stools in small quantity.
1149. Painful stiffness in the spinal column with heaviness and stiffness of the legs.
1158. Stitches in the back and left shoulder-blade.
1160. Drawing, tearing and cutting between the slouder-blades.
1175. Stitches in the neck and shoulder-blades.

Finally he rightfully quotes Dr. Koch's remark (Noack and Trinks. Hom. M. M.).

"Carbonate of lime has no direct relation to any one single organ, but produces a morbific effect upon certain systems, namely, upon such as by virtue of their organic structures either cover other organs, or form canals and cavities, the membranous and serous. It especially acts upon the mucous membranes, the fibrous and osseous system, nervous system, serous membranes and upon the venous (but also upon the lymphatic) system."

From this it is evident, therefore, that it becomes one of the most important remedies in diseases of reproduction.

Thus *Calc. carb.*, 3 trit., one grain morning and evening, was given.

Every other day ablution of the whole body in the room, with water of a temperature of from fifteen to eighteen degrees (R.), and walking about of the patient with the assistance of her friends.

*As early as fourteen days afterwards the improvement was remarkable.* Not only the dry cough, but also the fever decreased from day to day. After the course of a month the head did not require to be supported any longer. Pain in the back upon pressure only. Can walk around in the room without assistance. Mind more lively and active. Upon the upper part of the body and both arms, as well as at the nape of the neck, a slight eruption, somewhat itching, has shown itself within a short time.

Now *Silic.* 30, every second day, five globules, till the end of May, when patient could take walks out of doors again.

Of the disease nothing remained except that the head was carried bent down somewhat, but in case of an energetic will of the patient, it may be presumed that in this respcct, even, improvement is still possible.

Mention must also be made of *Calc. phosph.* The role it plays in scrofulous products is evident. We know that, besides carbonate of lime and chloride of sodium, *Calc. phosph.* preponderates in the lymph or the serous portion of the blood of scrofulous persons; we know, further, that the milk of scrofulous (tuberculous) cows contains seven times more phosphate of lime than other milk.* This surplus of saline salts is not accidental, and may, probably, be made use of by homœopathic therapeutics, as well as the fact that the abuse of Mercury reflects the entire picture of scrofulosis. *Calc. phosph.* so far as we know, has been justly recommended by French authors only, against chronic swelling of the tonsils, no doubt mostly upon a scrofulous bottom.

* Clark refers scrofulosis to an overloading of the general constructive material with phosphate of lime.

Heyne, of Beckum, praises *Calc. phosph.* 12 (to be given from three to four days every fourteen days) in tumor albus.

One word more of *Calc. acetica.* Dr. Hofrichter (Prague) calls it, as *Spirit. calc. acet.*, or as trituration of 1 : 100, or 1 : 10, repeated several times a day, the principal remedy in infantile diarrhœa. The principal symptoms, which, in his opinion, urgently demand its application are: inclination to looseness of the bowels and diarrhœa; diarrhœa with prolapsus ani; diarrhœa of scrofulous infants during dentition; in short, those cases of infantile diarrhœa described under the head of "softening of the stomach and intestinal tract" (gastromalacia). The diarrhœa sets in without any noticeable cause; the copious discharges rapidly following one another, according to the violence of the disease, consist of watery mucous, now greenish, flocculent stools, the cadaverous or characteristically sour smell of which, characteristic of the flatus also, soon communicates itself to the garments and bed-linen, and thus continually contaminates the atmosphere; at the same time slight fever, burning of the hands and soles of the feet, continual and intense thirst, loss of appetite, rapid emaciation of the whole body, and especially of the face, which assumes an aged look; continuous restlessness, tossing about; wailing and crying; pale, dry skin; sensitive elastically distended abdomen; occasional vomiting; scanty, pale urine, or easily disturbed sleep with eyes half closed (A. H. Z., 43, 11).

## CALENDULA OFFICINALIS.

### GENERALITIES.

"It promises to become a useful remedy in glandular diseases; the physiological proving, though aphoristic, already gives a few hints. Especially, it was recommended and used against scrofula by Tournecort, against bubo by Franc. Valleriola; against induration and carcinoma (scirrhus) of the mammary glands by Rudolph" (Dr. Reil, N. Z. f. h. Kl., 2, 9).

In developed scirrhus, carcinoma of the mamma and uterus, as well as in cutaneous cancer.

## CARBO VEGETABILIS.

### GENERALITIES.

"When in acute as well as chronic diseases the vital forces are nearly exhausted, the circulation begins to flag, a condition that reflects itself externally in cyanosis of evil omen; when the vital temperature sinks to a minimum, and the distress of the patient, whose mental capacities are mostly undisturbed, reaches its maximum; when all motions are expressive of the last smouldering vital spark; when we despair of all reaction, the effect of this truly magic remedy still surprises us, now and then."

### CLINIQUE.

### 1. (XLVIII.) *Atrophia.*

With the above words Dr. Hilberger, of Trieste, introduces a few interesting clinical observations on *Carb. veg.*, from which it is plainly visible when this remedy is indicated.

1. A feeble boy, 9 months old, whose mother while nursing him, became a victim to cholera, from this moment on suffered from diarrhœa that had lasted several months and seemed incontrollable. Though it had, finally, begun to abate somewhat, yet the little fellow did not pick up in the least, and the picture of atrophia infant. more and more developed itself. The child, emaciated to a skeleton, got into such a state of weakness that all capability of motion ceased, complete aphonia set in, and it could not take nourishment any more. Pulse small, scarcely perceptible, *the body cold.* Only the power of sight did not seem to be lost, just as a feeble breathing seemed to be the only sign of life left. For eight days it remained in this condition. For the sake of experiment, and more on account of the friends, I gave remedies which, however, were all fruitless; (*Sulph.*, *Arsen.*, *China*, &c.), finally, I administered two doses of *Carb. veg.* (6), and to the greatest surprise of all, as early as the next day, the child's voice returned, the temperature rose, and it was convalescent after receiving the remedy for fourteen days, and now is a lively and strong boy.

2. (XLIX.) *General Scrofulosis. Broncho-pneumonia.*

A child, æt. 2, who in the first year of life, had fortunately recovered from hydrocephalus, was attacked by whooping-cough, epidemic here the winter previous. For three weeks the disease took a tolerably favorable course, when on taking cold, pneumonia of the right side and an intense bronchial catarrh developed themselves additionally. The upper portion of the lung had already become somewhat emphysematous, the characteristics of the whooping-cough disappeared forthwith, but on the other hand, an extraordinary and continuous dyspnœa, mucous rattling, audible at a distance, even, and intense fever set in. In spite of all remedies (*Acon.*, *Bryon.*, *Sulph.*, *Phosph.*, *Tart.*) no improvement had taken place, and eight days afterwards the patient was in almost a dying condition. The skin cold, face bloated and cyanotic, extremities swollen, expression of the face corpse-like. Breathing so rapid that one could not distinguish the number of respirations. Excessive distress. The ominous wringing of the hands and the dull glances, looking out for help, of the child, who had its full consciousness, enlisted the strongest sympathy. Pulse could not be felt. Nothing but death by suffocation could be looked for now every hour. However, I gave the child one dose of *Carb. veg.* 6, and left two doses for the night. When I called the next morning, I scarcely credited my ears to hear that already after the first dose, half an hour afterwards, after so terrible an aggravation that the child was believed to be dead, more comfort set in. Upon the second dose the remedial aggravation had likewise appeared, but much weaker, and afterwards the dyspnœa decreased considerably, the pulse rose, the expression of the features became brighter. Improvement continued now for five days, when in consequence of stormy weather the child had a relapse, and the same sad phenomena reappeared. Upon *Carb. veg.*, an entirely similar reaction followed again, from which time on the child recovered slowly upon the administration of *Baryt. carb.*, which I always have seen act beneficially in similar cases, *when such affections appeared in scrofulous individuals.* The child now enjoys complete health.

## CARBO ANIMALIS.

### GENERALITIES.

Dr. Weiss takes a considerable quantity of beef or veal of which the fat is properly removed, adds bones amounting in weight to a third of the weight of the former, and burns the whole to coal in a common coffee-drum. After cooling, the coal is pulverized, and two and a half ounces thereof are mixed with two drachms of sugar, and of this mixture as much as the size of a pea, taken dry into the mouth and swallowed with a little water, against *inveterate and obstinate indurations of the glands.*

Healthy persons who take this remedy, are said to get knots in the mammæ, induration and swelling of the parotis and acne in the face, all of which affections, however, gradually disappear again.

According to Dr. Reil, a more rapid and energetic effect upon the glandular system is ascribed to animal than vegetable coal (Rust's Magazine, Bd. 22, 198).

Animal coal, on account of its peculiar relation to the glandular system and skin deserves the name of an antiscrofulosum with more right than vegetable coal. Especially the transition of scrofulosis into scirrhus would require the use of *Carb. animal.*, also the change of a benignant suppuration into a malignant ichorous discharge, and the presence of hard, painful glandular swellings. *Carb. veget.*, undoubtedly, manifests its curative effect, where pathological conditions are dependent upon a predominant venosity. Now, since many persons afflicted with scrofula, show such a predominance of the veno-vascular system, and especially torpid scrofulosis rests upon venous hyperæmia, *Carb. veg.*, also, ought to be made use of, especially, if burning pains accompany scrofulous affections.

Finally, let us not forget the great importance of *Graphites* in the therapeutics of scrofulous conditions, and that *Graph.*, though taken from the inorganic world, very much resembles the two kinds (*Carb. animal.* and *veget.*) of coal. For this reason we treat next on *Graphites.*

## CARBO MINERALIS—GRAPHITES.

### GENERALITIES.

*Graphit.* seems able to effect an improvement in the (crasis of the) blood. Many scabious, impetiginous, and dry exanthemata of the skin are cured by *Graph.* It is just the blood insufficiently oxidized, such as characterizes scrofulous individuals, that profits by the administration of *Graph.*, which has been used with benefit against highly developed forms of hydrops (hydrocele). It is no contraindication that *Graph.* is a remedy suitable to the female sex, and, at the same time, acts as an antiscrofulosum. Of the latter affections, two especially come within the sphere of its curative action: ophthalmia,* accompanied by photophobia and predisposition to hordeola, with simultaneous fissured eruptions around the mouth and nose; and impetigo of the hairy portion of the head, or herpetic eruptions upon various parts of the body of scrofulous youths. An affection related to herpes, its most intense expression, so to say, we find among women in the chronic ulcers of the foot with burning pain. In short, scrofula, in connection with an herpetic constitution, is the most appropriate field for cures with *Graph.*

*Dryness of the parts affected* (hence, burning pain, which manifests itself, for example, in ophthalmia, by acrid tears) is a symptom never absent where *Graph.* has helped. Here belongs, also, the often exceedingly obstinate constipation, very characteristic of *Graph.* *Graph.* resembles *Arsenic.*, with which it shows more points of contact (even in that form of gastralgia of the most violent kind, which is accompanied by vomiting and thirst), than *Iron*—a fact which might occasion surprise at the first glance.†

In common with the veg. carbon (*Carb. veg.*), the mineral (*Graphit.*) has the antiflative action. It cures (though not so often) the annoying distension of the stomach by gases, especially when such are found in females of sedentary habits. The accumulation of gases leads to real strictures, and in con-

---

* Especially in chlorotic, anæmic subjects, with simultaneous itching of the lid-edges, and a sensation of heaviness of the lids.

† Compare, also, the cure of Atrophia infant. by Arsenic. and Carb. veg.

sequence thereof to gastralgia of a periodical character (*e.g.*, at 4 A.M. and 4 P.M., &c.).

From this we see that *Lycopod.*, also, is not a very distant relative to *Graph.*, not to mention that *Lycopod.*, probably, surpasses *Graph.* in its bearing upon the phenomena of the herpetic constitution. In order to comprehend this existing connection, we must return to the genesis of herpes, which owes its origin in so many cases to suppressed activity of the skin (to a hypercarbonization of the blood).

In common with *Silic.*, *Graphit.* bears relations to the nutrition and plasticity of the skin; on the other hand, however, it does not mature abscesses as *Silic.* does.

This reminds us of another peculiarity of *Graph.*, which it has in common with *Silic.* in an eminent manner, to restore suppressed secretions, especially (venous) hemorrhages; while the secretions restored by *Silic.* directly refer to the sweat upon the skin of the feet. *Graph.* and *Silic.* cure fissured, withered ulcerous affections. Hardness of hearing (upon a scrofulous bottom) has also been removed by both. We must adhere, hence, all the closer to the differential momenta, according to which *Silic.*, more than *Graph.*, has direct relations to processes combined with suppuration, and alone deserves the name of a gland-remedy, and, above all, of a bone-remedy.

But there are still more remedies which have indications similar to *Graph.* Among these belong *Acid. nitri.*, an excellent remedy in scrofulous ophthalmia. *Acid. nitri.* is indicated in fissured, easily bleeding, and little secreting eruptive affections, in cases of chronic laryngitis (like *Graph.*), in cough, with a rough and dry voice; it is an ear-remedy (after scarlatina), and presupposes almost a similar constitution, as do *Graph.*, *Arsen.*, *Silic.*, and *Lycopod.*

However, a finer difference seems to lay in this, that *Nitr. ac.* corresponds more to the sycotic dyscrasia (condylomata, gonorrhœa, and gleet). *Graph.*, more to the scrofulo-herpetic contamination of the blood. Coarser differences are with *Graphit.* constipation, with *Acid. nitri.* diarrhœa. *Graph.* produces hemorrhages (similar here to *Iron*). *Acid. nitri.* arrests them. In regard to suppurating glands, *Acid. nitri.* is similar to *Silic.* Finally, no relation to the liver is known of *Graph.;* many, on the other hand, of *Nitr. acid.*

Scrofulous children, more than others, are subjected to hemiplegia of the face, though the occurrence may rarely happen by itself. Here, besides *Graph.*, the curative action of which has been proved (Kafka), *Caustic.* and *Petroleum* come under consideration. *Caustic.*, however, distinguishes itself forthwith by its antirheumatic virtues, suits, hence, in scrofulo-rheumatic affections; while *Petrol.*, aside from the similarity mentioned, has the following in common with *Graphit.*: "Scrofulous and rhachitic affections, itching herpetic eruptions, eruption on the head, hardness of hearing and deafness (from paralysis of the aural nerves), itching and swelling of the scrotum, and herpetic eruptions between scrotum and thigh. Cracked and fissured skin of the hands."

How, then, are we to distinguish *Graphit.*? For our purpose it suffices to know that, in doubtful cases, we may follow up *Graph.* by *Petrol.*, if constipation, already mentioned as a characteristic of *Graphit.*, does not forthwith decide for the one or the other remedy.

Finally, we could ask, What scrofulous affection does *Graphit.* cure, which is not also cured by *Sulph.*? We know that *Sulphur* suits decidedly more in scabious, *Graphit.* in herpetic eruptions; that, secondly, *Graphit.* presupposes more the peculiarities of the female sex, *Sulph.* more those of the male; boils, panaritia, suppurations of the tonsils, arthritic and rheumatic affections point to *Sulph.* alone, while eruptive disease-forms marked by their locality (behind the ear, at the scrotum), and such as are sufficiently characterized by their essence (erysipelas, the return of which *Graph.* is said to prevent, psoriasis palmaris, mentagra), allow of no other selection than that of *Graphit.* In short, *Sulphur* has a more extended sphere of action in the pathological processes characteristic of scrofulosis than the mineral coal.

*Graphit.* is also a coryza remedy. Kafka recommends it against ozæna scrofulosa, in case of purulent and offensive nasal discharge, ulcerated nasal openings, blood-streaked mucus on blowing the nose, smell as from burned hair, intense catarrh of the pharynx, with the sensation as if the food had to be swallowed over a lump, with simultaneous roughness and rawness of the throat.

According to Rosenberger, cases of coryza exhibiting the *herpetic character*, are suitable for *Graphit.*

## CAUSTICUM.

### GENERALITIES.

When speaking of *Calcar. carb.*, we have already mentioned the place which *Caustic.* holds within the series of antiscrofulosa, and content ourselves with enumerating the scrofula-symptoms pointing to *Causticum:*

1. Scabious eruptions, Scabies florida.
2. Stitching itching, with burning and redness after scratching.
3. Burning on all places touched.
4. Nightly agglutination of the eyes; frequently dark-colored webs and fiery sparks before the eyes.
5. Otorrhœa.
6. Obstruction of the nose, and continuous coryza.
7. Yellowish, discolored, sickly complexion, with yellowish temples and palish-blue lips.
8. Pressure in the stomach from eating bread, even; much inclination to empty eructations.
9. Large abdomen in children; chronic constipation; frequent, but unsuccessful attempts at stool.
10. Involuntary escape of urine.
11. Chronic hoarseness and weak voice; feeling of soreness in the chest and larynx.
12. Strumatous swelling of the thyroid gland.

Thus we have an imposing series of scrofula-symptoms. Aside from *Calc. carb.*, we probably think of *Hepar* and *Mercur.* as analogues, with which it has, moreover, great chilliness and profuse sweats in common.

We have to consider, hence, all the more the few differential momenta. *Caustic.* is, so to say, the *Rhus* of the mineral kingdom, and, besides, acts more upon scrofulous affections with burning spread over a surface (Scrofula cutanea). It has not the specific relation to pus that *Merc.* and *Hepar* have, which we mentioned.

The true significance of *Caustic.*, in general, and to scrofulosis particularly, will, probably, become more clear by presenting a few of the exceedingly practical remarks of A. C. Clifton, of Northampton.

According to them, *Caustic.* has proved itself efficacious in scrofulous and rheumatic ophthalmia, especially if constipation existed simultaneously; in general dryness of the skin; in rheumatic paralysis of the left side of the face, in consequence of cold northwest wind, and in rheumatic prosopalgia of the same side.

Moreover, the same author cured with *Caust.* fistula lacrymalis, and fistula in ano (by its internal and external application).*

*Caustic.* was very efficient in chronic rheumatism with swelling and stiffness, with contractions of the tendons (in getting up after sitting the tendons in the knee-joint as if too short), with stinging and tearing pains, especially in scrofulous subjects, though it frequently required *Calc. carb.*, *Silic.*, and *Sulphur* to finish the cure.

*Caustic.* helped in psoriasis palmaris, also in otorrhœa of children, when a dry eruption behind the ear and around the nose existed at the same time. The author found this remedy very efficacious in constipation of children, especially if accompanied by enuresis nocturna; in case of a dry, unhealthy skin, upon which every small wound passes into suppuration (a principal criterion of scrofula); in dryness of the rectum, with vehement contraction of the sphincter ani, on account of which children were compelled to retain the stool for several days.

It is, also, a valuable remedy in laryngeal cough; in phthisis, if the cough appears in the morning, and is accompanied by tickling in the throat, and difficulty in raising the mucus; in hoarseness and aphonia.†

Its relations to the uro-genital system, the local atonic affections of which it cures, enable us almost alone to distinguish between *Caustic.* and *Graph.*, with which it has no fewer than the following characteristics in common:

---

* Staphisagr. 30 (one dose every evening), is also praised in fistula lacrymalis (A. H. Z., 77, 79).

† In acute cases Causticum 3; one drop every two hours.

1. Antiscrofulosum;
2. Constipation;
3. Burning and itching pains;
4. Eruption behind the ear;
5. Psoriasis palmaris;
6. Hemiplegia facialis;
7. Chronic laryngitis; rough voice;
8. Dryness of skin; fissures;
9. Ophthalmia.

## CLEMATIS ERECTA.

### GENERALITIES.

"Regarding it the same holds good that has been said of *Calendula;* homœopaths saw satisfactory cures from it in swellings of various glands and in torpid scrofula" (Dr. Reil, N. Z. f. h. Kl., 1, 9).

"As regards the exanthemata, in which we are guilty of generalizing too much, *Clematis* seems to have been much neglected. It has proved itself efficacious especially in the pustular forms (papulæ, acne, sycosis). Here I have found it to be specific and exceedingly prompt in its action; much more efficacious than in eczema (impetigo, bullæ, ecthyma); in short, in the vesicular forms, in which it has also been recommended from different quarters" (Hirschel, N. Z. f. h. Kl., 2, 23).

Dr. Steus names *Clematis* among the cancer remedies (besides *Con.*, *Lycopod.*, *Sep.*, and *Sulph. ac.*) (N. Z. f. h. Kl., 4, 19).

Dr. Kallenbach praises the curative power of *Clemat. erecta* in tumors of the mammæ, with simultaneous affection of the whole mammary gland (otherwise not), especially if the pains are aggravated by west wind, cold weather in general, and during the night.

Dr. Weber corroborates the efficacy of *Clemat.* in such cases, saying that he had found it confirmed in a girl to whom he had given this remedy for soreness of both nasal openings.

v. Boenninghausen remarks upon this that the principal indication for *Clemat.*, in such glandular affections, is a burning, tensive, and itching pain, which is considerably aggravated, especially after *cold washing*, or cold, wet applications (Neunte Jahresvers. d. hom. Aerzte Rheinlands und Westphalens, 31 Juli, 1856. A. H. Z., 53, 12).

NOTE.—The testicle corresponds to the mamma.* We see now that *Clemat.* shows its action upon that also. From all this it may be seen that *Clemat.* suits better for grown-up persons; hence for the scrofula-forms more modified by increasing years, among which affections, finally, we may rightly count the scirrhous degeneration of the glands. At any rate, the remedy ought to be tried in affections of the skin and glands, with due observation of the indications above mentioned:

1. Torpidity of the trouble.
2. Aggravation from cold and wet.
3. Glandular organs affected, or the skin amid efflorescence of a papulous exanthema.
4. Burning, tensive, and itching pain in the part affected.

## CONIUM MACULATUM.

### GENERALITIES.

*Conium* has a more decided action upon the glandular system than *Cicuta*, belonging to the same natural family, which manifests its effects more in the nervous system. Not only the ancients, Dioscorides, Plinius, Avicenna, observed after the use of *Con.* the glands of healthy persons to grow smaller in size, but also more recent experiences have confirmed these facts. Especially do all agree in its pain-allaying action.

Dr. Kurz (N. Z. f. h. Kl., 2, 9) recommends *Con.* against periodical, nightly cough, if predisposition to scrofula sustains the cough. My own clinical observations corroborate these recommendations. *Con.* 3, a few drops in two grammes of alcohol. Of this from 2 to 3 drops from three to twelve hours (N. Z. f. h. Kl., 2, 14).

---

* For this reason abuse of Iodium occasions atrophia of the testicles, as well as of the mammæ.

The relations of *Conium*, says Dr. Hilberger, of Trieste, to glandular affections, and especially to the mammary gland, were already surmised by old school physicians. Physiological provings have confirmed these properties *de facto. The considerable hardness of an infiltrated gland, and the flying stitches resulting from its pressure upon the nerves*, form a principal indication for its administration. It develops its effect most likely by causing a reaction in the compressed, and hence relaxed nervous and vascular ramifications, and in this manner brings about the resorption of the softening tissue, without, however, being capable of altering the dyscratic character itself.

The N. Z. f. h. Kl. 2, 21, recommends *Con.* 6 against photophobia and presbyopia, already manifesting itself in early years.

In the same journal, Bd. vi (x), 24, a cure by *Conium* is mentioned; a few noduli, resembling hard beans, in the left mamma, with a slight short cough (in a young lady æt. 25), were resorbed upon the use of—

℞. Conii macul. fort. gtt. iij.
Sach. lact., gr. vij (0, 5).
M. f. p. d. dos. t., No. xii.—Two powders daily.

Dr. L. Battmann (of Grossenhain) deems *Con.* (2) the most specific remedy in suppuration of the mesenterial glands, and in support of his opinion quotes the report of an interesting case (A. H. Z., 54, 21).

## CLINIQUE.

### 1. (L.) *Affection of the Nervus laryngeus inferior*,

Consisting in a clapping sound in the larynx, in a scrofulous boy æt. 13, with previous spasmodic pressure in the region of the ligamenta glottidis. Dr. Schwenke supposed pressure upon the n. vagus, in consequence of glandular swelling, and cured the trouble by *Con. mac.* 6 rapidly and permanently. Allopaths had given the same remedy before without result (A. H. Z., 49, 19).

## DULCAMARA.

### GENERALITIES.

Characteristic remedial action (according to Altschul): suppurating, *wetting*, herpetic eruptions; *vesicular* eruptions, with a yellowish, watery liquid; glandular swellings, and induration of the glands; bad effects of taking cold, especially from wet, cold weather; sudden hydropical swelling of the body (hydropical dyscrasia).

### CLINIQUE.

1. (LI.) *Scrofulosis.*

In the long account of suffering of a boy, æt. 1¼, in whom, as usually, accompanied by obstinate, sour diarrhœa, vomiting, knotty distension of the abdomen, subsequent cough, and furunculous eruptions, &c., an exceedingly high grade of general scrofulosis and atrophia developed itself, Dr. Buerkner (N. Z. f. h. Kl., 3, 9) marks out two periods. After the malady, in spite of the most careful dietetic as well as therapeutic treatment of the child, had already become very severe; when the child, emaciated to a skeleton, with a shrivelled, wrinkled skin, covered on the back, buttocks, and legs, with furunculous, hard, red knots, lay in bed, which it soiled several times daily by excessively fetid, thin discharges, not crying any more, but hoarsely moaning the whole time; a pemphigus, the bullæ of which partly had the size of a pigeon's egg, broke out over the whole body, amid the most distressing restlessness. Against this, though with no hope of success, *Dulcamara* 1 was prescribed every two hours; a remedy which the writer remembered to have seen recommendeded against this disease-form. Almost from the very moment of its application, improvement set in in the general condition of the child; it became more quiet; the diarrhœa grew less; sleep came on; and when, five or six days afterwards, upon the continued use of the remedy in a higher dilution, even the pemphigus blisters, to which, at the beginning, a few fresh ones had been added, began to heal up, the whole condition was so changed, that one could again entertain hope for the child, given up long ago. And, in fact, from this date on, recovery evidently progressed without any further medicine; yet an unexpected occurrence was again to endanger the results so laboriously obtained. After matters had been comparatively well, and the child had improved considerably, an intense inflammation of the knee-joint developed itself. The left knee was thickly swollen, painful, tense, and red; violent fever; great restlessness, and a return of diarrhœa accompanied the localization of the scrofulous process. The development into suppuration and gonarthrocace seemed inevitable. However, a few doses of *Silic.* 12 quickly arrested the evil, and after that time the recovery progressed so rapidly that from six to eight weeks afterwards the patient was completely well, and could run about again upon healthy legs.

## EUPHRASIA.

### GENERALITIES.

We can easily name a dozen remedies which are said to cure scrofulous ophthalmia and its concomitant phenomena. At what time, hence, is *Euphras.* to be applied? It corresponds apparently to a simultaneous sycotic (condylomatous) dyscrasia, and has been given against condylomata after *Thuja* had been used in vain.

Euphrasia has, moreover:

Inflammation and redness of the eyes.

Inflammation and ulceration of the edges of the eyelids, with headache.

Spots, vesicles, and cicatrices on the cornea; also opacity of the same.

Watering of the eyes, especially in the wind.

Much secretion of mucus in the canthi, with nightly agglutination of the lids.

Profuse coryza with discharge of acrid tears and photophobia.

### CLINIQUE.

#### 1. (LII.) *Spots upon the Cornea.*

Dr. Jackson as long as forty years ago, has recommended this remedy against spots upon the cornea. In a boy who suffered from a very violent and obstinate scrofulous ophthalmia which left spots of considerable size on the cornea, this remedy alone was efficacious (Brit. Journ. of Hom., 1850, Jan.).

### 2. (LIII.) *Opacity of the Cornea.*

In April, 1851, I observed the rapid curative effect of *Euphras.* 1, daily one drop in three tablespoonfuls of water, four days in succession, in a young female badger dog, against a severe blennorrhœa of the conjunctiva of the right eyeball, and pterygium, which, departing from the inner canthus, spread over nearly the whole transparent cornea. The pathological formative process ceased forthwith, and the pterygium disappeared in the shortest time without any further local application. The most prominent symptoms were: intense redness of the eye, swelling of the lower lid, increased mucopurulent secretion, nightly agglutination of the lids, and photophobia (A. H. Z., 44, 16).

NOTE.—Dr. Lobethal, on the contrary, says that in scrofulous ophthalmia the effect of *Euphras.* is uncertain, and appropriately assisted by the internal use of *Cannabis* and *Nitri acid.*, and in case of severe photophobia by *Rhus* 1.

He thinks that in catarrhal ophthalmia *Euphr.* is of acknowledged efficacy, a reason for which it is kept officinally in all drug stores.*

We also believe that *Euphras.* in the most pernicious form of scrofulous ophthalmia, can never render superfluous such remedies as *Calc. carb.*, *Acid. nitri.*, *Mercur.*, *Arsenic.*, &c. It can claim here, consequently, but the name of a so-called intercurrent remedy.

## FERRUM.

### GENERALITIES.

If Iron were of benefit in anæmia alone, we could not use it much in scrofulosis; however, it cures those diseases coincident with dropsical conditions, and, from this view, it is an antiscrofulosum.

---

* Aus den Verhandlungen des Vereins schlesischer hom. Aerzte, in Breslau, A. H. Z., 76, 10.

We name (according to Rueckert's industrious compilations) the following confirmed indications:

1. Relaxation and weakness of the entire musculature and emaciation, weakness of digestion, coldness of the extremities.

2. Anæmia under the mask of plethora and congestion, accompanied by a whitish color of the mucous membranes.

3. Pulmonary tuberculosis, especially in young, florid subjects with a remarkable erethism of the vascular system, inclination to congestion toward the chest. But we will remind here of the property of *Iron*, in larger doses, to occasion hemorrhages, a reason for which allopathic physicians do not give it in tuberculosis with inclination to hemorrhages.

4. Aphonia, very distressing.

5. Chronic, watery diarrhœa in children, usually soon after eating and drinking, *without pain and effort*, mostly containing undigested substances.*

*Iron* is the remedy, also, indicated after previous abuse of *Iodine* (likewise after *Arsen.* and *China*), and what scrofulous patients have not already been overfed by *Iodine* (or a compound thereof) when they are transferred to us from allopaths?

The Monatsblatt to the 82d vol. of the A. H. Z., presents a very interesting contribution to the action of *Iron*. There we find an essay by Dr. E. Seitz (of Buer, near Osnabrueck), which shows that a great number of strumata decidedly grow in size and are produced by the use of *Iron* preparations (confirmed in Virchow's Jahresbericht of 1868, Bd. 1, Abth. 2, S. 287).

"Very similar relations," continues Seitz, "exist moreover, with regard to scrofulous glandular swellings, and every objectively observing physician may convince himself that with some scrofulous children the submaxillary glands grow larger and more painful after the administration of *Iron* preparations"† (Allgem. med. Central-Ztg., 1870, 103).

There exists scarcely a more direct appeal to give *Iron* in a homœopathic preparation against such glandular hypertrophies. Allopaths can, probably, best quiet their conscience by giving *Iodide of Iron*, in place of *Iron*. For *Iodine* as surely

* Calc. carb. or acet., Phosphor., Arsen., are more frequently administered against this affection as the expression of a scrofulous trouble.

† Calc. carb. or acet., Phosph. and Arsen., are more frequently indicated in this affection as an expression of scrofula.

reduces the size of the glands (especially of the gl. thyreoidea) as *Iron*, according to Seitz, increases it.

## HEPAR SULPHURIS CALCAREUM.

### GENERALITIES.

Coinciding, as a general thing, with the action of *Sulphur; Hep. sulph. calc.*, on account of its combination with lime, still more acts upon the lymphatic and glandular system, and especially moderates plasticity. Hence its curative action in pathological processes with pseudo-membranous deposits (croup). Secretions of the skin and mucous membranes are excited by it, as well as exudations of serous membranes more rapidly resorbed by it. Like *Sulphur* itself, *Hep. sulph. calc.*, affects disturbances dependent upon prevailing venosity. All this insures to it a prominent position among the antiscrofulosa.

*Hepar* has shown itself useful in the following forms of scrofula-dyscrasia:

1. In abscesses, the maturing and suppuration of which are hastened under its influence.
2. In moist and wet tinea.
3. In panaritia, in which *Hepar* in alternation with *Silic.* renders surgical interference superfluous.
4. In inveterate glandular indurations, which are brought to suppuration or resorption by it.
5. Its curative action is indubitable in scrofulous ophthalmia, in which it acts all the surer the more pure the habitus scrofulosus presents itself in its totality.
6. In scrofulous, purulent otorrhœa.
7. In angina membranacea, in croup and pseudo-croup. They, as is well known, cannot always be distinguished from each other during life, as long as real membranes are not coughed up. *Hep. sulph.* soon changes the dry, harsh, and crowing cough into a loose one. We do not always succeed in this with *Spong.*, which is still more used in the treatment of croup. The torture of emetics is spared to children, treated homœopathically, on account of the certainty with which our remedies, among which *Hep. sulph.* belongs par excellence, bring about a crisis.

8. Again *Hepar* recommends itself in relapses of amygdalitis. We find chronic enlargement of the tonsils as an unmistakable expression of existing scrofulosis. Every cold settles there. After *Bellad.*, the reduction of the tonsils which have grown still larger, hesitates sometimes; then *Hep.* ought to be given.

9. Against ulcerated corners of the mouth.

10. In ophthal. neonator. (simultaneously with the external application of *Acid nitri.* See that).

11. In febrile flowing coryza, when the flow becomes very easily arrested, especially in scrofulous and rhachitic children; if hoarseness or a hollow rough cough appears in addition (Kafka).

12. In ozæna scrofulosa (Kafka).

*Mercurius* is the remedy with which *Hepar sulph.* could be confounded most easily. *Mercur.* within the domain of scrofulosis has almost all the therapeutic virtues of *Hepar sulph.* Hence we shall have to fall back upon the total characteristics of both, in order not to commit any mistake. Yet this is not to be understood as if both, now and then, were not in place, one soon after the other (in a similar manner as *Lycopod.* may immediately be given after *Calc. carb.*), *e. g.*, if the improvement obtained by *Hepar* comes to a standstill (see note to LIV and LVI).

Both remedies have in common:

1. Pain as from being bruised.
2. Excessive sweats.
3. Inflammatory swellings of the glands.
4. Acne rosacea.
5. Scrofulous ophthalmia and otitis.
6. Inflammation and suppuration of the tonsils.
7. Great flow of saliva.
8. Dry cough.
9. Symptoms of rheumatismus acutus; inflammatory erysipelatous redness and pains.
10. Leucorrhœa.
11. Panaritium.
12. Coryza, with copious discharge of an acrid fluid.

DIFFERENCES.

*Hepar sulph.*

1*a*. Difficult stool as from inactivity of the intestines.*

*Mercurius.*

1*b*. Bloody mucous stools, excoriating the anus. Greenish, slimy (bilious) stools. Tenesmus. Dysentery.

*Hepar sulph.*

2*a*. Has many more specific relations to the exudative process of the larynx.

*Mercurius.*

2*b*. *Mercur.* is never used in croup so often; in hoarseness and pseudo-croup we find *Hepar* indicated.

On the contrary, *Merc.* more than *Hep.* in cases of angina which are occasioned by swelling (formation of abscesses) of the tonsils, inflammation of the uvula (accompanied by copious flow of saliva).

*Hep. sulph.*

3*a*. Efficacious in mercurial dyscrasia.
Long-continuing or retarded suppuration.
Festering, easily ulcerating skin; putrid, fetid, carcinomatous ulcers. Hair falls out very much.

*Mercurius.*

3*b*. Various manifestations of syphilis fall within its therapeutic sphere.
Nightly inflammatory pains of the bones. Inflamed swollen suppurating glands.
Highest degree of emaciation.
Ulcerated, whitish-dentated, detached gums, looseness and falling out of the teeth. Fetid salivation.

---

* In certain cases Hepar even is to be considered as a remedy in dysentery; yet we read in the proving of Hepar more of whitish and muco-sanguinous diarrhœa, or sour-smelling and whitish discharges.

Inflammatory swelling and suppuration of the inguinal glands (bubo venereus).

*Hepar sulph.*

4*a*. *Hep. sulph.* corresponds more to the torpid form of scrofula.

*Mercurius.*

4*b*. In scrofulosis erethica et florida.

*Merc.*, moreover, cures also the following affections which cannot be reached by *Hepar*.

*a*. Epilepsia (Trinks).
*b*. Zona with violent burning-itching at night (Schroen).
*c*. Icterus and cutaneous œdema after scarlatina.
*d*. Nervous fever with pain in the region of the liver, diarrhœa, and easily-bleeding gums.
*e*. Typhus abdominalis, in its first stage, with tenderness of the liver (status biliosus et pituitosus).
*f*. Gastric and scorbutic stomacace.
*g*. Glossitis.
*h*. Atrophia mesaraica, with a large abdomen of the infants, soft stools, and hectic fever (see Arsen).
*i*. Gonorrhœa, dysuria, stranguria, hæmaturia.
*k*. Balanitis from suppressed gonorrhœa (Trinks).

We briefly repeat that the affections cured by *Merc.* presupposes a greater participation of the organs connected with the production of bile than is the case with *Hepar*. The latter better corresponds and is more suitable to the infantile organism, and for this reason, even, better fitted to be a more many-sided remedy in scrofula than *Mercur.*, inseparable from the idea of syphilis.

### CLINIQUE.

#### 1. (LIV.) *Scrofulous Ophthalmia.*

A. N., æt. 7, of a very well-marked scrofulous habitus.

The left eye intensely inflamed; the sclerotica of a violet-reddish color; the cornea turbid and dusty-looking; the eye watering profusely; the lower lid swollen; great photophobia.

High potencies of *Bellad.*, *Calc.*, and *Hep.* had no effect.
Feb. 21st. *Hep. sulph. calc.* 3, trit. four doses.
" 23d. Pain decreased.
" 24th–28th. One dose daily. As early as on the 25th, the ulcer is evidently smaller and flatter; and, on March 2d, a complete cure has been accomplished.*

NOTE.—"Scrofulous ophthalmia, in which the lids are reddened, swollen, and agglutinated, accompanied by ulcers on the cornea, require *Hepar sulph.* as their principal remedy" (sometimes beneficial in alternation with *Mercur.*,—*Hyd. præcip. rubr.*) (A. H. Z., 77, 10.)

2. (LV.) *Croup.*

Anton Scholz communicates a cure of croup (probably of pseudo-croup only) with *Hep. sulph*, of which he gave one grain (4th trit.) every hour: "All danger was removed as by magic, and I had good reason for praising *Hep. sulph.* as an excellent remedy" (A. H. Z., 24, 13).

3. (LVI.) *Ophthalmia Neonatorum.*

Rueckert does not doubt that *Hep. sulph. calc.*, this efficacious remedy in catarrhal and scrofulous ophthalmia, especially in intense affection of the Meibomian glands (Kl. Erfahr. 1, 235 and 271), now and then, will act favorably also in ophth. neonat. (N. Z. f. h. Kl., 5, 12); and we read on page 79, Bd. 77, of the A. H. Z., of a very bad case, in which the cornea was pouched out, all the soft tissues of the eye were thickly swollen and of a spongy appearance, accompanied by a terrible purulent discharge and photophobia, which was treated with the best result by *Hep. sulph.* (in the morning) and *Merc.* 3 (in the evening).

4. (LVII.) *Eczema of the Head.*

Mr. N., a government officer of high rank, asked advice with regard to his children, who exhibited a well-marked

---

* Ein Beitrag zur Frage ueber die Hochpotenzen von Dr. Kallenbach in Goerlitz. A. H. Z., 30, 7.

scrofulous habitus, and suffered at times from glandular swellings and acne, as well as from numerous small boils.

The whole family went to Kreuznach, since the father, likewise scrofulous, suffered from a chronic conjunctivitis of both eyes; he also took the baths, and afterwards drank the water of the Elizabeth spring.

During the drinking-cure small vesicles had already appeared upon the head; first at the occiput, which soon spread over the vertex and synciput as far as to that portion of the forehead free from hair. The vesicles had become larger and larger, formed thick crusts, which discharged a moisture, and, upon drying up, thickly covered the portion affected, so that but one yellowish-white crust was visible, which detached itself in form of light scales and lamellæ, covered the clothing and floor, and caused violent itching, especially at the parts covered with hair. The hair itself seemed sickly, died off, and fell out more and more.

A Parisian physician, who declared the trouble to be Eczema rubrum, and a consequence of the use of the Kreuznach springs, since it had been present once before, prescribed, without result, *Rhus tox.* and *Merc. sol.*, after which the discharge became more copious. *Graphit.*, which counteracted the latter effect, and produced more dryness; *Sulph.*, *Phosph.*, *Clematis*, which comforted much; *Laches.*, which subdued the redness, did most without curing definitely, however; Sulphur-Amidine baths, which acted favorably upon the thickness of the crusts; *Dulcamara.*

When Hirschel saw the eruption it was confined to the scalp, and presented the form well known as eczema impetiginosum. *Hepar sulph.* was selected, 1, in view of the antidotal relation to the effects of *Iodium* and *Bromium* contained in the waters of Kreuznach, which, at all events, had awakened the dormant scrofulo-dyscratic conditions, and brought them to the surface; 2, in view of the existing scrofulous foundation of the cutaneous affection itself; and 3, in consideration of the peculiar form of the eruption, the "moistening soreness," "inflamed cutaneous surface," "puriform discharge," "crusty character," of which, as well as its "secretion of a whitish-bubbly liquid," "its itching and itching-gnawing," together with the "falling out of the hair," are distinctly recorded in our M. M.

He gave the remedy in the 3d trit., one grain of it morning and evening, combined with the use of baths, each containing two ounces of *Hep. sulph.*, of which, however, on account of the advanced season, but three could be taken; forbade the use of all others, even the most innocent washes or softening oils, in order to keep the head perfectly dry, and ordered the strictest diet. After eight days already a complete arrest of the trouble manifested itself; since the eruption did not spread any further, the moisture decreased, and the itching grew less. Six weeks later the cure, in its main feature, was completed. The eruption dried off more and more; the crusts separated easier, grew thinner and thinner, the cutaneous redness, at the place of the detached crusts, more and more disappeared. The subsequent crop, in place of the crusts, showed but scales which easily detached themselves; small, dry noduli, in place of the filled vesicles. The hair fell out more and more. Only at the occiput it remained; and here, also, the most intense itching was experienced, against which glycerine was allowed to allay it. At first the vertex healed up, next the synciput, then the occiput, and, latest of all, the right parietal surface, upon which the most intense redness of the skin had been observed. When the *friseur*—two months too late—brought the wig ordered, he was surprised that it had become unnecessary, since all parts of the scalp were healed, and the hair in a healthy growth. Only one spot made a stubborn resistance; for, after the affection of the scalp had healed, the eruption spread from the right parietal bone over the right ear, and crept from the right auricula into the meatus audit. This affection was removed by *Hep. sulph.* 2 within four weeks, so that the whole cure required the time of ten weeks.

Besides *Hepar sulph.*, *Mercur. sol. Hahn.* 2 was interponed but two or three times when the reaction following upon *Hepar* came to a halt. Then discharge and aggravation* always set in, but forthwith upon the reapplication of *Hep. sulph.* the improvement progressed in a most decided manner.

---

* This aggravation, no doubt, could have been prevented in the most simple manner by selecting a higher dilution in place of the 2d trit.

### 5. (LVIII.) *Scrofulous Ophthalmia.*

Dr. Genzke communicates a very interesting cure with *Hep. sulph.* (A. H. Z., 55, 10), in a boy, æt. 10, who suffered from highly developed scrofulous ophthalmia. Photophobia, gush of tears, considerable opacity of the cornea, and whatever else characterizes such an inflammation were present. *Hep. sulph.*, 2d trit., one grain every evening, removed the inflammatory stage within four weeks; afterwards *Aurum* 3 the opacity of a high grade.

### 6. (LIX.) *Swelling of the Axillary Gland.*

The same author applied with the best success *Hep. sulph.* 2, three times a day, against an affection of three months' standing. The trouble had begun with violent tooth and face-ache, which were accompanied by drawing pains in the whole body, especially in the arm, in addition to which the right axillary gland began to swell and became painful. Loss of appetite. Sleeplessness. Presently enormous swelling of the axillary gland, which renders any motion of the arm impossible. The gland was firm, here and there studded with pus-pustules, discharging a viscid pus. Inunctions of all sorts, and continued for months, and warm poultices had proved themselves useless; only periodically the pus-pustules broke, the swelling itself successively increased in hardness and circumference. Within eight days we succeeded in scattering the swelling by *Hepar sulph.*, and in simultaneously removing the morbid general symptóms (A. H. Z., 55, 20).

Note.—We see from the reports, or rather cures, presented that, as we have said above, *Merc. sol.* frequently insures and completes the effect of *Hep.* Upon the whole we may say *Merc.*, with its indication of *thin* stools, suits, *cæteris paribus*, in the first stage, that of irritation; *Hep. sulph.*, with its pathogenetic effect, *hard* stool, in the second, that of paralysis, to express it in a somewhat extreme manner.

# IODIUM AND ITS PREPARATIONS.

## *A.*—IODIUM PURUM.

"Iodium est avec Silicea le meilleur médicament de la scrofule."—Jousset.

### GENERALITIES.

Notwithstanding many contradictory statements, it is a fact that Iodium, in its physiological action, has a specific influence upon the glandular system. At the beginning and after small doses the secretions of the glands are mostly somewhat increased, but even if intense salivation has sometimes been observed after Iodium, it is, as a general thing, much less the case than with Mercury, and more dependent upon individual irritability. On the other hand, two other important phenomena have been noticed to appear after the use of Iodine, namely, atrophia of the mammæ and testes. It was found, however, in autopsies that other glandular structures even, such as the mesenterial and suprarenal glands, had grown smaller after the continued use of Iodine, as well as that the fat and connective tissue had been consumed.

However, experience *ex usu in morbis* much more decidedly argues for the specific action of Iodium upon the glands. Hypertrophies of the most various glandular structures, as well as of other formations differently constructed, tuberculosis and scrofulosis have always been, and will ever continue to be, the curative domain of this potent remedy. (Dr. Reil, N. Z. f. h. Kl., 1, 9.)

The remark of Dr. Knod v. Helmstreit, that Iodium has proved itself efficacious against mercurial ulcers, salivation and stomacace of scorbutic nature, may also be mentioned here, because the scrofula-process is frequently complicated with the affections named.

Dr. Schweikert is of the opinion that among the inhabitants of regions, the springs of which contain Iodine, struma is occasioned by the physiological action of the frequent use of Iodium; hence, in a similar manner as we see it with regard to Calc. carb., which possesses the power both of causing and curing goitre.

Iodine, as we have seen above, cures the affections provoked by the abuse of Mercury; but, since the latter represent a pathological picture very similar to scrofulosis, Iodine will be, hence, of decided usefulness in scrofula. Thus Iod. recommends itself against glandular swellings with induration; ophthalmia and aural diseases; scrofulous bubo; large, chronic strumata;* laryngitis; tracheitis; angina membranacea; tumor albus, even of an inflammatory character, and with violent pains and suppuration; against inveterate cutaneous diseases (impetigo scrofulosa).

### CLINIQUE.

#### 1. (LX.) *Cure of Struma.*

A female servant, æt. 28, since her fifteenth year, has suffered from a considerable enlargement of the thyroid gland. Since eight days, there is a noticeable swelling of the left thyroid gland, already enlarged, which increased so considerably that she scarcely could breathe any more. She talked so laboriously, and her respiration was so difficult and noisy, that she had to hold head and neck entirely stiff, and distort the facial muscles of the left side. Upon the thyroid gland (of the left cervical region), already much enlarged, a swelling as large as a man's fist is to be seen, which is but little movable, oviform, and presses upon larynx and trachea. Iod. 3, in pellets, two pellets every two hours. After four days, condition the same. Iod. 20, for three days, without any perceptible improvement; from this time on, however, the swelling decreased so much from day to day, that on the tenth day of treatment the portion situated at the right side of the trachea had entirely disappeared, and there could be found but a somewhat hard swelling, as large as a pigeon's egg, at the left.

* Iodium acts beneficially only in struma lymphatica, less so in st. cystica, but is absolutely harmful in st. aneurismatica, such as develops in women during the act of parturition (Altschul).

Respiration entirely good; can remain in every bodily position* (A. H. Z., 60, 11).

Swelling and induration of the glands, emaciation with ravenous appetite, inclination to tubercular meningitis, all point to Iodium. It corresponds to caries, to pleuritic exudation, phthisis, and tubercles; suppuration, with and without caries. According to Jousset, injections of Iodine (the pure or diluted tincture) prevent the appearance of hectic fever; it moderates suppuration, and unexpectedly often effects a cure. On the other hand, we read in the "Universal-Lexicon der pract. Medicin und Chirurgie," in the article on scrofulosis, written with much industry and professional knowledge: "In case of tubercular degeneration and suppurating abscess, the results of Iod. have been naught. Frequently the effects were harmful and fatal in cases of scrofulous cachexia, which were accompanied by febrile symptoms and emaciation."

In the A. H. Z., 46, 8, we find the following warning example against traditional doses of Iodine:

"A girl, æt. 18, ruddy, and well developed, consulted a physician on account of a swelling of the throat, a so-called 'saddle-throat' (Sattelhals). He prescribed an Iodine salve and Tr. iodii in increasing doses up to fifteen drops three times a day. When I was called to see the girl, six months afterwards, she had changed so that I scarcely could recognize her. Her form was withered, the bosom had disappeared, her face was of an ashy pallor, and around the eyes blue rings had formed. She complained of a large number of troubles, especially of oppression, dry cough, palpitation of the heart, loss of appetite, pressure in the stomach. The menses, previously regular, and at first failing to reappear after taking the medicine, had afterwards appeared all the more copiously, and since that time she had almost from every three to four days, a discharge of a thin watery blood from the vagina. The situation of the patient was a dangerous one. At any rate, by the clumsy experiments with Iodine, the blossom of a youthful life is destroyed forever."

Where, then, is to be found the true, curative sphere of

* Dr. Lobethal cannot do without a salve of *Kali jodat.* (05 : 90, 00) in the treatment of large lymphatic strumata.

Iodium? The following case may present the answer to this question.

2. (LXI.) *Asthma Laryngeum.*

A child, nine months old, suffering from atrophia mesenterica, underwent treatment for this trouble. Emaciation has not yet reached the highest degree; abdomen large, legs thin, stools irregular, now constipation, now diarrhœa. In addition there were troubles from teething. Upon the administration of *Calc. carb.* and *Sulphur*, alternately every other day, the child improved rapidly. But fourteen days afterwards convulsions set in, which presented the following symptoms: Sudden rigidity of the body, bending back of the head, tight closing of the hands, lips growing purple and, in connection therewith, the appearance as if the child were strangling; respiration momentarily suspended; dry heat of the skin, and frequent jerks and starts. The attack appeared usually when crying or coughing, and at waking up.

In consideration of the periodical heat of the skin, *Aconit.*, and afterwards *Bellad.* was given, but although the heat disappeared, the spasms nevertheless remained as before. *Ipecac.*, as well as *Hep.* (the latter on account of the peculiar sound of the cough, reminding one of croup) effected nothing; after *Zinc. met.*, it is true, no general and fully developed spasm reappeared, but still momentary constriction of the larynx. The sound of the cough, the glandular affection and the general emaciation, as well as the irregular stools, led me to give *Iod.* Upon its use the attacks soon became weaker, and finally ceased entirely. Under the continued application of this remedy, the child is now strong, fleshy, and healthy.

In a second case of asthma laryng., *Iodium* did the same good service; in a third it only helped in alternation with *Sambucus* (Dr. Seybel, Aschersleben, A. H. Z., 50, 15).

In croup of scrofulous children, which likewise has its asthma laryng., *Iodium* deserves the greatest consideration, and it seems almost as if many cures with *Spongia*, which is related to the former, in most cases had appertained to spurious croup (without formation of membranes) only. Otherwise, how could such facts as the following find an explanation?

C. A. Tietze, 1839, treated fifteen children affected by croup with *Acon. Spongia* 30, and *Hep. sulph.* 3. Not one of them died. One year afterwards five died out of six. (An ominous symptom was the entire absence of cough.)

From the experience obtained, *Iodium* is, hence, a sovereign remedy against croup. Before we make mention of the surprising cures effected by it, we will briefly cite the following symptoms from its pathogenesis: "Intense disturbance of respiration. Oppression with pains when taking a full breath; stronger and more accelerated pulsation of the heart, and smaller and more frequent pulse. Difficulty of breathing in the throat. Soreness with whistling in the throat. Inflammation of the trachea, hoarseness; sensation as if something had lodged in the larynx that could be removed by hawking. Titillating and tickling (in the throat). Increased secretion of mucus. Viscid mucus. Dry cough with oppression. Heaviness in the chest, &c.

"Great lassitude. Weariness. Great prostration. Weakness of the muscles.

"Distress. Anxiety. Oppression in the chest."

Trinks knows of but two kinds of croup, the acute and the torpid. *Iodium* is specific to both; he needs no *Aconit.*, rarely *Hepar sulph.*, and ascribes the favorable results obtained to the continued administration of the specific remedy in repeated and increased doses, if the intensity of the disease is not broken by weaker doses, and there is no qualitative change.

### 3. (LXII.) *Croup.*

A boy, æt. 5, very scrofulous, with many and large cicatrices on the neck, occasioned by glandular suppurations, was attacked by croup. On the second day of the sickness, which presented all the symptoms of croup in the highest degree, "attacks of suffocation, sawing sound, dry, crowing cough, soundless voice with intense fever, &c.," patient received *Iod.* 2, two drops every hour, besides, oatmeal poultices. For three days no change in his condition; at the fourth, decrease of the synochal fever with simultaneous eruption of a rash on the throat, back, and chest which, on the day following, covered arms and feet also. The croupous symptoms, not so intense any more, increased on the next day, more and more. *Iod.* 2, up to five drops, every hour. At the eighth day decrease of the croup-symptoms, only the cough remains dry, and has a metallic sound up to the eleventh day, when it becomes more loose and solvent. *Hepar sulph.* 3, one grain every four hours, removed all the remaining symptoms (Hom. Vierteljahrschrift, 3, 2, Trinks).

### 4. (LXIII.) *Iodine Vapors successfully applied in a Severe Case of Croup.*

BY DR. W. ARNOLD, OF HEIDELBERG (A. H. Z., 2, 19).

Membranous croup, by the specific remedies that homœopathy has given into our hands, is usually treated with such success as soon to remove all its danger. Though the cases which resist our method of treatment for a longer time, are rare, they yet occur sometimes; especially if the patient comes under our treatment after the disease has already lasted some time and has progressed considerably. In several cases of this kind, which partly had been given up by other physicians, I have successfully used *Iodium* internally. In a few other cases which resisted this remedy, even, and which would have prompted some physician to perform the operation of tracheotomy, I found myself induced to let *Iodium* act directly upon the mucosa of the respiratory organs; and I have always seen the best result from this procedure. *Not only were the lives of the three children in whose cases I saw myself compelled to apply Iodine vapors, saved, but they recovered completely, i. e., no subsequent diseases of the respiratory organs occurred.*

In one of the three cases the croupous inflammation had confined itself to the larynx; in the two others bronchial croup was plainly marked. The effects of the Iodine-vapors could soon be recognized by the fact that after the cough had become somewhat moist, some mucus intermixed with membranous fragments was expectorated shortly afterwards, which brought some relief, though very slight at the beginning. However, upon the repeated application of the vapors, the cough became more and more loose, and, aside from a mostly very viscid mucus, and amid the strong efforts of coughing or vomiting, the children threw up smaller or larger pieces, and sometimes longer shreds of the pseudo-membrane. Upon the frequent use of the *Iodine*-vapors and under the continuation of the expectoration mentioned, the distress and dyspnœa of the little patients decreased rapidly; they fell into a sleep which, though lasting but a short time at the beginning, became longer and more quiet after each expectoration brought about by the paroxysms of cough. In this manner the danger had disappeared within sixteen hours in the one case in which the croupous inflammation was confined to the larynx, in the two others within from forty to forty-eight hours.

The plainly perceptible effect of the *Iodine*-vapors consisted, hence, in changing the character of the cough, making it more moist, in the detachment of the membranous formations and the relief of respiration dependent thereupon.

The *modus operandi* simply consisted in dropping a few drops of the second decimal solution up to several drops of the strong *Iodine tincture* into a flat vessel with boiling water, and letting the child inhale the vapors; which was accomplished by holding its head over the steaming water or closely to it.* The process, according to necessity, was repeated oftener or less frequently from two to six hours. At the commencement the vapors appeared to be agreeable to the children, for they tried to come near to the steaming vessel. Afterwards the effect seemed to be disagreeable to them, for two of the children offered resistance against their application, after relief of the symptoms had already set in.

### 5. (LXIV.) *Laryngitis exsudativa* (*Croup*).

BY DR. SCHLOSSER, OF MUNICH (A. H. Z., 49, 20).

M. S., a boy, æt. 2½, for three days hoarse, has a dry cough, which daily increases under increase of the fever.

July 14th, 1853, about 1 A.M. the child wakened up with a violent attack of suffocative cough, which lasted several minutes, afterwards it went to sleep again, but at dawn was again disturbed in its slumber by a dry, hoarse cough, accompanied by great difficulty of breathing.

---

* Nowadays we would use one of our common inhaling apparatuses. Thus I have applied locally not only *Iod.* but also *Graph.*, *Brom.*, *Hep sulph.*, &c.

On the next morning fully developed idiopathic laryngeal croup. Intense fever, dry skin, hoarse rough voice, short laborious, sawing respiration, with frequent, dry, and barking cough returning in paroxysms. Pharynx intensely reddened, the larynx painful on touch. The symptomatic picture did not leave any diagnostic doubt as to the trouble being laryngeal croup.

*Aconit.* 3, three pellets pro dosi, and *Iodium* 3 gtt. j ; in Sach., lact., 1, 0, m. f. p. To be given alternately ; one hour *Aconit.*, the other of the *Iodine*-powder as much as will lay on the point of a pen-knife, with a little water.

After a few hours, considerable amelioration in the attacks of cough and difficulty of breathing set in ; six days later he was completely cured, though no exudative membranes had been removed by vomiting, so that a complete resorption has to be presumed.

In conclusion Dr. Schlosser says: Though this favorable termination is usual with our curative method, every cure of genuine croup deserves, nevertheless, to be recorded, since under allopathic treatment most of the children affected by it die, and the cure of this disease may possibly induce the thinking portion of old-school physicians to turn to the study of homœopathy ; especially, such of them as cannot befriend themselves with the barbarous, though unreliable method of the local internal cauterization with Nitrate of Silver, and have found the emetic and local-antiphlogistic methods ineffective.

### 6 and 7. (LXV and LXVI). *Two Cases of Angina Membranacea cured by Iodine Vapors.*

BY DR. KIRSCH, OF WIESBADEN (A. H. Z., 57, 13).

One of the children, a girl, æt. $2\frac{1}{2}$, had already been treated without success allopathically with emetics for four days, and an older child of the same family had shortly before died of croup (at the eleventh day of the disease).

When the second child was attacked by the disease, the physician had declared, that it seemed to set in with the same violence. In fact, all the symptoms of croup had reached so high a degree in the surviving child, that there was but very little hope for resorption of the exudation and recovery.

*Aconit.* and *Brom.* had not the slightest effect. Now from fifteen to twenty drops of the first alcoholic dilution of *Iodium*, to a saucerful of hot water (put over an alcohol-lamp) were allowed to vapor off near the child. It became stupefied, but did not improve in the least, and was near suffocation. Now the third trituration of Iodium was used for the development of the vapors. Improvement set in as early as after the first inhalation, and within forty-eight hours, during which time five such inhalations had been taken, the child had recovered.

If from this report, rightly remarks Dr. Kirsch, the efficacy of Iodine-vapors becomes evident, the proof is also presented thereby, that the curative power of a remedy does not lay in the quantity of the substance, but that often only a smaller portion of a medicine renders it a curative remedy, and that the expansion of the molecules is of no little importance.

Another child, ten months old, also took inhalations of Iodium (3d trit. two grains in a saucerful of water, vapored off over an alcohol-lamp). The vaporing off of such a quantity lasted half an hour. Repetition in two and a half hours. After three inhalations the cough became looser. Afterwards inhalations every six hours, *Aconit.* as an intercurrent remedy against the fever. The croup terminated with the appearance of coryza.

We interpone the remark here that cases of croup have terminated fatally in which neither in the larynx nor trachea a trace of exudation was found on autopsy. These cases (according to Dr. Schlautmann and Professor Niemeyer), are said to have been occasioned by a collateral œdema of the laryngeal muscles, and in consequence thereof by paralysis glottidis.* From this the inefficiency of the remedies, otherwise helpful, may be explained, as well as the curative power of drugs not employed usually.

According to Kidd (Brit. Journ. of Hom., April, 1859), *Iodium* is thus far the most efficacious remedy against diph-

---

* See A. H. Z., 20, 57. Vortrag des Herrn Dr. Schneider aus Magdeburg: "ueber den croup."

theritis. He advises to give large doses of it, frequently repeated, also inhalations of pure *Iodine*, vapored off in the room. We take notice of this view without indorsing it. It is possible that in those cases in which Iod. (even in a homœopathic dose), helped, diphtheritic croup was present. It is suspicious in Dr. Kirsch's case that two children of one and the same family were sick with croup. Genuine (non-diphtheritic) croup, so far as we know, is not contagious.

In No. 12 of the N. Z. f. h. Kl., Dr. Lobethal (Breslau), reports upon the administration of Iodium dilutions in "malignant cases of membranous croup," and continues as follows: "But also in acute catarrhs of the larynx and in inflammation of it, in hoarseness of singers from taking cold (not in aphonia), as well as in chronic irritation of the larynx with hoarseness in the evening, especially in persons who were scrofulous when children, dilutions of *Kali iodatum*, or still better, of *Iodium*, are of great value."

He sees between Kali iod. and Iodium a relation similar to that between the mother-tincture of a remedy and its dilution.

## *B.*—OLEUM JECORIS ASELLI.*

"As regards its local-specific action, cod-liver oil is a very good symptomatic remedy in scrofulosis and tuberculosis. But in tuberculosis it is by no means a curative drug in the true sense of the word."—KAFKA.

It would be one-sided were we not to take notice of cod-liver oil in our treatise on anti-scrofulous remedies. Because it has been greatly abused, does it therefore possess no virtue? The fact alone that it contains *Iodine* ought to point to its importance in scrofulosis.

Moreover, have not many of our invaluable remedies been taken from the ocean? Chloride of Sodium, Sepia, Iodium, Bromium, Spongia, and even the Carbonate of Lime, obtained from oyster-shells, all have important and, we may say, in many respects unknown relations to the processes of scrofulosis.

* The unpurified (brown) C. L. O , according to A. Vogel, is preferable to the purified white.

"An extended sphere of action," Dr. Madden says, in a paper on Ol. jec. asell., read before the Brit. Hom. Society, in 1848, "is conceded to it, especially in scrofulous diseases and all their kin, and above all where the osseous tissue suffers, as in rhachitis, caries, spina ventosa, &c. In diseases of the mesenterial glands and atrophia dependent thereupon, it is not any less efficacious. Scrofula, as is well known, appears in individuals of two different bodily states; individuals of the one look fresh, fleshy, and fat; those of the other pale, lean, emaciated, and cachectic. The remedy is especially efficient in the *latter*, but only exceptionally in the former."

According to Dr. Madden, *Iodine* even is effective only in lean scrofula, and not in the fat.

In osteomalacia, atrophia mesenterica, and phthisis pulmonum, especially in tuberculosis, when the tubercles have not yet softened entirely, cod-liver oil proves its efficacy. According to Bennett's* observations, it surely cures chronic cutaneous diseases, scrofulous ulcers, and ophthalmia.

The administration of cod-liver oil, limited though it be, can be justified from the standpoint of homœopathy all the more, as the symptoms which the oil occasions in the healthy correspond with those of Iodine as recorded by Hahnemann. Kopp was the first to point to the fact *that Ol. jec. aselli is efficacious in those cases in which physicians prescribe small doses of Iodine.* And Falkner found that the oil contained $\frac{1}{40000}$ portion of *Iodium*, a quantity which is equal to that in our 4th or 5th dilution. The mineral springs of Kissingen, Kreuznach, Nauheim, Salins, likewise act as antiscrofulosa by virtue of their homœopathic contents of Chlorine, Iodine, and Bromine.

But since *Iodine* does not show itself as efficient as the oil, the oily menstruum must share essentially in its curative power. Observations have taught us that those continually handling fatty substances are fleshy and free from scrofula. It has been endeavored to demonstrate by experiments in what manner the fat exerts a beneficial influence upon the body, and it has been found that it forms a kind of emulsion

* Dr. Hughes Bennett has exhausted in his work (1841) everything that can be said on C. L. Oil.

with albumen, in which emulsion every molecule of fat is inclosed in a kind of albuminous capsula.* Since the chymus contains much albumen and acid, the acid becomes neutralized by the admixture of bile, among the constituents of which fat and soda belong, and the fat in connection with the albumen forms the chylus. The most recent researches have demonstrated the importance of the oil for the animal economy, from which the great benefit of the cod-liver oil in scrofulous diseases becomes evident, the origin of which depends upon deficiencies in the process of digestion, in which the emulsion does not possess the normal quantitative character. Some have proposed even to diminish the scrofula-diathesis by inunctions of the body with various kinds of oil.

Ol. jec. aselli, Dr. Madden concludes, has hence two important bearings upon the organism:

1. On account of the oil itself; and,
2. On account of its contents of Iodine.

The physiological effect of the former does not interfere with the pathogenetic (therapeutic) effect of the latter, in consequence whereof the remedy, besides being very digestible, is very appropriate for the diseases mentioned above.

Though Dr. Madden may probably expect too much of cod-liver oil, he yet gives us important hints for its application, the remark, by itself, being of great value, that the scrofulo-plethoric habitus does not correspond to it, a thing that many allopathic physicians do not seem to know, for to them cod-liver oil is the true antiscrofulosum *à tout prix*. As regards the digestibility of the cod-liver oil, it is plain from what has been said, that not every stomach will bear it; and why not? This much is sure, however, that some children evince no aversion to it, while others show the greatest disgust for it.

It would be interesting to ascertain whether scrofulosis is to be found among the inhabitants of Greenland and the Esquimaux, who count all kinds of oils among their delicacies, and do their share in using inunctions. However, we may infer its exemption with regard to the polar regions, *à priori*, from the fact, previously mentioned, that the disease belongs to the temperate zone.

---

* Sunderlin—Behrend's Vorlesungen, Bd. 5, 220—is of the opinion that in scrofulosis the *chylus* contains too much *albumen*.

It is, probably, not superfluous to quote here a remark from the A. H. Z., 46, 6:

"*Test of cod liver oil.*—If we dip a strip of copper or brass into pure cod-liver oil, the metal is not changed by it. If, however, the cod-liver oil is adulterated with vegetable oil, the metal assumes a green color, if after dipping it into the oil, we expose it to the air."

In the Dublin Medical Press, Oleum cocos is recommended by Thompson as one of the best antiscrofulous remedies, which is equal in effect to cod-liver oil.*

We add the data of a chemical analysis of cod-liver oil, according to Dr. Jongh:

| | Cod-liver Oil. | | |
|---|---|---|---|
| | Black. | Brown. | White. |
| Oleic acid, gaduine, and two other substances as yet not definitely determined, . . . | 69,951 | (59,106?) 50,106 | 74,033 |
| Margaric acid, . . . . . . . . | 16,145 | 10,121 | 11,758 |
| Glycerine, . . . . . . . . | 9,711 | 9,075 | 10,127 |
| Butyric acid, . . . . . . . . | 0,159 | 9,075 | 0,074 |
| Acetic acid, . . . . . . . . | 0,125 | 9,075 | 0,046 |
| Choleic acid (Acides felliniques et choliniques), | 0,299 | 0,062 | 0,043 |
| Bilifuolin and bilifellinic acid, . . . | 0,376 | 0,445 | 0,263 |
| Substance soluble in alcohol, . . . . | 0,038 | 0,015 | 0,006 |
| Substance insoluble in water, alcohol, and ether, | 0,005 | 0,002 | 0,001 |
| Iodine, . . . . . . . . . . | 0,0295 | 0,041 | 0,037 |
| Chlorine, with some bromine, . . . . | 0,084 | 0,159 | 0,149 |
| Acid. phosph., . . . . . . . . | 0,054 | 0,079 | 0,091 |
| Acid. sulph., . . . . . . . . | 0,010 | 0,086 | 0,071 |
| Phosphorus, . . . . . . . . | 0,0075 | 0,0114 | 0,021 |
| Magnesia, . . . . . . . . | 0,004 | 0,012 | 0,009 |
| Soda, . . . . . . . . . | 0,018 | 0,068 | 0,055 |
| Lime, . . . . . . . . . | 0,082 | 0,012 | 0,009 |
| Waste, . . . . . . . . . | 2,569 | 2,603 | 3,209 |
| | 100,000 | 100,000 | 100,000 |
| | | 91,000? | 100,002 |

(E. T.)

* But we remind the reader of the fact that the black, as well as the white C. L. O., contains acetic acid, by virtue of which such a reaction may take place.

Hence, cod-liver oil, according to the opinion of all authors, acts by virtue of its contents of *Iodine*, *Bromine*, *Phosphorus*, and *Chlorine*. But, as we see from the above table, all those substances exist in truly infinitesimal proportion, if compared to the quantity of fat, indifferent in its nature.

Dr. Weil, without hesitation, calls cod-liver oil "a natural homœopathic dilution of oil in fat."* However, the recommendation of cod-liver oil in cases of scrofulosis, with emaciation, speaks eloquently and decidedly in favor of the idea that we have to do with a homœopathic preparation, not only as regards the quantitative proportion of *Iodine*, but also, and above all, as regards its therapeutic action; for the effect of large doses of *Iodium* upon the healthy consists in *atrophia* of all the glandular tissues, as well as other structures; in short, in emaciation.

We meet with an entirely similar view in the excellent pathologico-therapeutic study of Kafka, "Anæmia, or Blood-pallor" (A. H. Z., 59, 24).

He considers cod-liver oil to be "*a homœopathic dilution of an Iodide of Phosphorus*," and for this reason deems it to be appropriate only to definite disease forms, corresponding to its physiological sphere of action.

Since, however, the glands, the skin, the mucous membrane of the respiratory organs, and the osseous system, are the principal parts upon which Iodine, as well as Phosph., have a decided effect, its therapeutic application, in his opinion, extends only:

1. To all forms of scrofulosis and tuberculosis of the glands, especially if the hyperæmic and inflammatory processes have run their course, and a chronic swelling has remained.

2. To all forms of scrofulous cutaneous diseases which produce exudations, such as eczema, impetigo, pityriasis rubra, tinea, favus, prurigo, &c., as well as in that degeneration of the cutaneous follicles which is known by the name of cutaneous tubercle.

3. To all chronic catarrhal processes of the organs of respiration, *e.g.*, of the nose, larynx, pharynx, trachea, bronchi, &c., which accompany scrofulosis and tuberculosis.

---

* Anleitung zur Krankenpflege, von Dr. Weil, S. 102.

4. To all scrofulous diseases of the bones, joints, periosteum, as well as to tuberculosis of the bones.

5. Also rheumatic affections, so far as they lay within the sphere of action of *Iodine*, especially if they are connected with chronic exudations in the joints, between the muscles, or in the subcutaneous cellular tissue, are suitable for the application of cod-liver oil.

Moreover, the opinion of those therapeutists deserves notice who attribute an essential share of its action to "*the admixture of decomposing liver-elements*," which can be found in all kinds of cod-liver oil.

"There has been a good deal of debating, A. Vogel says, as regards the active substance proper of cod-liver oil. Some believe that by its large amount of fat it simply act as a means for respiration; others search for its efficacy in the traces of *Iodine* and *Bromine;* still others, finally, in its *fatty acids*, and the admixture of *decomposing liver-elements.*"

Since experiments with pure fat as well as with small doses of *Iodine* and *Bromine*, did not produce the results desired, the latter view seems probably the most tenable.

It yet remains for us to utter a word of warning as regards the external use of cod-liver oil. By the application of compresses saturated with it, we very easily succeed in the rapid removal of tinea-eruptions on the head; but *these* very exanthemata by no means are local processes, but the expression of scrofulosis coming to the surface. A sudden suppression occasions an obstruction and exsiccation of the innumerable springs, the contents of which now make a retrogressive movement; or, more scientifically, the liquid pathological products are resorbed and deposited in the interior; meningitic and pneumonic processes are developing, or in the most favorable instance, hardness of hearing, otorrhœa, diseases of the eye, &c.

To our treatise on the physiological and chemical peculiarities of cod-liver oil we finally attach the appeal to try it in the form of inhalations in croup. In almost all grave cases of genuine croup it has thus far been necessary to employ several of the most approved remedies. Since, however, Bromine, Iodine, and Phosphorus, above all, belong to the latter, and all of these are contained in the cod-liver oil, it is possible that by virtue of this combination of the specific antiscrofulous elements, a great preventive and curative power results with regard to the disease named.

### CLINIQUE.

#### 1. (LXVII.) *Coxarthrocace.*

Dr. Knod v. Helmstreit has published (in Hufeland's and Osann's "Journal der pract. Heilkunde, Bd. 74, Mai") several cures of chronic rheumatism and coxarthrocace by cod-liver oil.

A boy, æt. 6, in consequence of a fall on the knee, was affected by coxalgia, which, on account of improper management, reached the suppurative stage, so that the femur was entirely driven out of the hip-joint, and the leg became shortened. The abscess opened anteriorly, and daily produced from four to six ounces of pus of such acrid nature as to inflame the parts to which it adhered for a time. The boy had a severe hectic fever, was exceedingly weak, emaciated to a skeleton, and inevitably seemed to be doomed to die. For fear that cod-liver oil would still more disorder the appetite, already very poor, it was first applied in injections (1½ ounces twice a day). Later the child took two, and four weeks afterwards three tablespoonfuls daily. Improvement was perceptible as early as after six days, and progressed without interruption. The fever gradually disappeared, suppuration became benign and less copious, the pains ceased, and strength returned; in short, the fistulous ulcer had healed completely after the use of cod-liver oil for six months and a half.

## *C.*—KALI HYDROJODICUM.

The action of *Kali hydrojod.*, Schoeman says, in general agrees with that of *Iodine*, but nevertheless undergoes unmistakable modifications by the combination of the latter with Kali.

It is used by the old school:

1. Against *all forms of scrofula, swellings of the glands,*

*scrofulous blennorrhœa, chronic skin diseases upon scrofulous bottom.* Scrofulous ulcers. Scrofulous ophthalmia (Magendie); against pannus and leukomatous obscuration of the cornea (Chelius); induration of the mammæ and hypertrophy of the lacteal glands.

2. Against *goitre* — struma lymphatica — allopathic text-books recommend from 2 to 5 grains three or four times daily.

It seems absolutely necessary, however, to illustrate by an example what value is to be placed upon recommendations from this side, especially as it is to be the principal aim of this small essay to expose the dangers contained in the orthodox allopathic therapia; to show how, in fact, the efficacy of the remedy, correctly selected, is only too often annulled by the senseless adherence to large doses.

"A man, æt. 62 (Goullon, Sr., writes, A. H. Z., 45, 5), very bilious, and suffering from gout since his youth, received of an allopathic physician Kali jod. (℈ij in ℥iv of water) against ischias, with the advice to take a tablespoonful morning and evening for weeks. About eight days afterwards a very suddenly increasing swelling of the whole thyroid gland appeared, with tenderness on touch and dyspnœa; he nevertheless was told to continue the remedy, and in the second week manifested all the symptoms of endocarditis: dyspnœa; fainting, with great exhaustion; violent, jerking, intermitting, and irregular beat of the heart and pulse; tensive pain across the chest; especially the right ventricle was affected, which at the same time gradually enlarged somewhat. Besides, loss of appetite and vomiting. Mercur. 2, in several doses, and Arsen., on returning aggravation a few days later, removed the trouble almost entirely. Sepia removed the remaining symptoms."

If the obnoxiousness of massive doses is demonstrated by the report of this case, the highly specific relation of *Kal. hydrojod.* to strumata, very correctly pointed out by the old school, is evident from the following communication of the same author, just as the very fact mentioned that upon the use of large doses of *Kali hydrojod.* intumescence of the glandula thyreoidea was observed, clearly enough proves such a specific bearing.

CLINIQUE.

1. (LXVIII.) *Struma.*

A young blooming girl feebly menstruated on account of a dry, oppressive, and painful cough, which had lasted for years, and was connected with heaving and whistling respiration, both troubles being dependent upon a large swelling of the thyroid gland, which pressed inwardly and downwardly; after a resultless administration of *Phosph.* and *Calc.*, received but four grains of *Kal. jod.*, in four ounces of water, half a table-spoonful morning and evening. As early as ten days afterwards the cough, and the symptoms connected therewith, had entirely disappeared, and the thyroid gland become smaller and soft, so that it did not occasion any further trouble.

Is not the truth of the homœopathic curative principle brilliantly set forth in these two reports? In the pathogenesis of *Kali jodat.*, swelling of the thyroid gland after large doses; according to clinical experience, decrease of the strumatous swelling after small doses.*

Finally, another example of the injuriousness of large doses.

A girl, æt. 13, took *Kali jod.*, a few grains morning and evening for several weeks against scrofulous ulcers, caries of the lower jaw, and a very malignant scrofulous ophthalmia with ulcers on the cornea. Under this treatment the ophthalmia was cured rapidly and permanently, and the ulcers improved so much as to form cicatrices, when she was attacked by pneumonia which rapidly passed into suppuration, and of which she died.

According to the above, *Kali hydrojod.* has a cumulative effect, similar to chloroform, which makes the person to be operated upon fall into a beneficial sleep, but which, above the effect desired, has already put many to eternal sleep.

The syphilitic bear *Kali hydrojod.* better than the scrofulous.

---

* We cannot omit the remark, however, that in the case mentioned the small doses were still not small enough; for we read at the close of the report of the second case: the patient, who felt entirely well, had lost flesh in a remarkable manner (during the administration of Kal. hydrojod.).

The sleeplessness of which patients complain, even after proportionally small doses of Iodide of Potassium, is worthy of notice.

## *D.*—FERRUM JODATUM.

### GENERALITIES.

Ferrum jodat. is indispensable also to us homœopaths in complicated scrofula. It accomplishes more here than the pure antiscrofulosa, such as Silicea, Phosph., Iod., Calcar., &c. One does well not to give it in infinitesimal doses. *Ferrum jod.* is indicated where chlorosis, rhachitis, and syphilis combine with scrofulous processes. It removes especially impetigo of the cheek, and eczematous exanthemata of the face and whole body.

### CLINIQUE.

#### 1. (LXIX.) *Hydrocephalus.*

A child who suffered from Hydroc. acutus in a high degree, and previously had been treated with Calomel and Jalappa, and fly-blisters to the head, was saved yet by *Ferr. jodat.* in the paralytic stage.*

Dr. Langheinz states having observed this specific curative power of *Ferr. jodat.* in from six to eight cases, when children, who are anæmic and poor in flesh, were attacked, or when such a condition had been produced artificially by previous antiscrofulosa (leeches, calomel, jalappa).

Rueckert in his attempt at utilizing the curative material obtained *ab usu in morbis*, gives as indication for *Ferrum: Hydrocephal. acutus, with large, open fontanels*, from which follows that the *iron* in the Ferr. jod. was probably more essential in the cases quoted above than Iodine.

---

* The diagnosis had been made out by Prof. Winter and another experienced physician of the University of Giessen (A. H. Z., 60, 19).

2. (LXX.) *Eczema of the Whole Body* (*E. rubrum*).

(My own observation.)

C. S., a small, fleshy, and very scrofulons boy, was brought to me with a general, moist, eczematous eruption which formed thick, dirty crusts on several places (temples, forehead). Extensive, circumscribed eczematous spots on various parts of the body; at the outer surface of the right lower leg a fiery-red, hot, and moist spot resembling raw-meat. Violent itching and ill-humor accompanied this characteristic eruption. *Graph.* and *Arsen.* caused the beginning of the improvement; but the crusts fell off in the course of fourteen days upon the use of *Ferr. jodat. sach.* (0, 03 triturated with 2, 0 Sach. lact., as much as will lay on the point of a knife). The presence of crusts resembling *bark* seems of some importance for the selection of *Ferr. jod.*

### *E.*—CALCAREA JODATA.

GENERALITIES.

Recommended by Vehsemeyer against struma and chronic hypertrophy of the tonsils. It corresponds to scrofulosis of an intense form. For those chronic scrofulous intumescences of the tonsils remain up to virile age, and frequently occasion intercurrent catarrhs of the larynx. Upon the use of *Calc. jod.* the swellings, the fissured appearance with the cup-shaped excavations of which is characteristic, decrease in size.

I have learned highly to appreciate the remedy in ophthalmia perniciosa of scrofulous persons, when *Calc. carb.* remained without effect.* *Calc. jodat.* undoubtedly has a great future.

### FOLIA JUGLANDIS.

GENERALITIES.

Negrier (Arch. gen. Fevr., Avr., 1850), praises walnut leaves in scrofulous affections. According to him, they produce

* The report of the respective case is to be found in the A. H. Z., 22 Mai, 1871.

diuresis, sometimes also diarrhœa, and especially affect the digestion, a statement which is confirmed by Cl. Mueller's experiments (Dissertat. inaugural. de jugl. reg. viribus. Lips. 1843). They are said to have less effect in diseases of the bones, than in affections of the skin, glands, and eyes (Z. f. h. Kl., 1, 1).

Besides Negrier, Miraut, Jurine, and Altschul corroborate the antiscrofulous effect of walnut leaves. Nasse recommends the remedy against helminthiasis, otorrhœa, and fluor albus scrofulosus; Hauser in cutaneous eruptions, tinea capitis.

Recently it has been used in hypertrophies of the tonsils and their chronic swelling (4, 0 of the extract to 30, 0 of aqu. dest., applied by means of a painter's brush).* Internally 0, 2 in 15, 0 of water, from ten to fifteen drops daily against infantile diarrhœa.

It has also been employed externally against spots upon the cornea.

In ophthalmic practice, I saw good results of the internal administration of Tinct. juglandis (1st or 2d dil.), against chronic blepharadenitis ciliaris with tendency to general vascular injection of the eyes.

## KALI AND ITS PREPARATIONS.

We should leave a great gap in our work, were we not to mention the salts of potash in our compilation of the antiscrofulosa. For Kali carbonicum is able to arrest incipient pulmonary tuberculosis; the latter, however, is the most intense expression of scrofulosis. The Chromate of Potash corresponds, as we soon shall see, to all the remaining, most obstinate manifestations of scrofula. The principal character of the Kali-preparations consists in the arrest of profuse and abnormal secretions, whether they appear as hemorrhages or purulent or serous secretions. Besides this we know that *Kal. carb.*, has an undeniable influence upon the heart (hence upon circulation), and that portion of the nervous system

* *Calcar. jodat.* (Vehsemeyer) or *Kali bichrom.* (Drysdale) are probably more specific.

regulating the activity of the heart. Otherwise the two preparations of Kali differ so much from another, as to induce us to speak of them separately.

## *A.*—KALI CARBONICUM.

### GENERALITIES.

We have already mentioned the importance of *Kal. carb.*, as regards the lungs; before, however, tuberculosis has fully developed, catarrhs of the nose and larynx precede it; our preparation corresponds, therefore, to these troubles of a definite and specific character. The chronic character and inclination to relapses, as in all scrofulous affections, stand out prominently even here.

Hence Kal. carb. cures dry coryza, which renders breathing through the nose impossible, but becomes fluent *upon walking in the open air, and returns in the room*, and is accompanied by a great deal of itching in the nose and secretion of a yellowish-green or bloody mucus; in other cases, a puriform mucous discharge, mostly from one side of the nose, and of an offensive smell; burning pain in the nose; sore, crusty nasal openings, even entire obstruction of the nasal openings; bluntness of smell; in the evening often intense, fluent coryza with frequent sneezing and headache, rough voice, a titillating sensation in the throat, which creates a desire for hawking and coughing, and the feeling of firmly lodged mucus (A. H. Z., 1 Febr., 1869).

"Kali, says also Kafka, is an excellent remedy in dry coryza with *complete hoarseness* and *aphonia*, in catarrh of the pharynx with the sensation of a plug in the throat; in nocturnal spasmodic cough and tussis titilans; in strangling and gagging which terminate in vomiting, especially in the morning." Graphit. also has the symptom of the "*plug*" when swallowing; Caustic. the symptom of hoarseness and aphonia.*

* STINGING pains, in many cases, indicate Kal. carb.

## *B.*—KALI CHROMICUM.

The Chromate as well as the Bichromate of Potash deeply affect inveterate scrofulous troubles, and it is just their obstinate character that furnishes a palpable indication for the administration of these remedies. For this reason they cure genuine membranous croup, ozæna, and such forms of coryza as by their long duration have almost become physiological processes, so to say. The hypertrophy of the tonsils, of no less chronic a nature, as well as the malignant forms of cutaneous eruptions, fall likewise within the curative sphere of these drugs. Suspicion of a combination with hereditary syphilitic causes render more sure the propriety of selecting them.

### CLINIQUE.

#### 1. (LXXI.) *Membranous Croup.*

A boy, æt. 8, with all the symptoms of membranous croup received *Tinct. Aconit.* and *Tinct. Iodii*, of each four drops in half a wineglassful of water, a teaspoonful every two hours alternately; besides a wet, cold towel across the chest and throat, renewed as often as it became warm.

The disease was not removed by these means; on the contrary some symptoms had grown worse, and, upon local examination, one could plainly see the upper part of the larynx covered with white and thick membranes.

In place of Iodine, *Kali chromic.* 1, two drops in four ounces of water, was given every three hours, alternately with *Aconit.* Since the skin was burning hot, the cold applications were continued with more energy. Four hours afterwards a piece of membrane as large as a finger-nail was coughed up. The fever decreased, and within four days several pieces of membrane, one more than three inches long and half an inch wide, were thrown up by the cough, and blood and bloody mucus were coughed up from four to five days, until the cough changed into a simply catarrhal one. After this remedy had been given for a week the boy could be considered cured. Wherever this remedy proved efficacious the mucosa of the nose became sore (from "The Hom. Times," by Dr. Bamberg, Berlin (XXXII) 9).

As regards the developing soreness of the nose, we deem it in place to remind the reader of a remark of Goullon, Sr. (during a discourse before the meeting of the Centralverein, August 10th, 1854). He observed scrofulous nasal crusts to develop after the cure of *genuine croup, which, as a general thing, he considers to be a scrofulous affection.**

Connected therewith is the recommendation of Chromate of Potash against the obstinate and intense form of chronic, dry coryza (upon scrofulous bottom).

### 2. (LXXII.) *Chronic Scrofulous Coryza.*

A young, apparently healthy girl, for several years suffered from ozæna and an affection of the throat. Syphilis had been the primitive cause. Continual discharge of a yellow mucus from the nose; the mucosa red and shiny; the bones not affected or tender. Dryness and rawness of the pharynx; its mucosa red, as if varnished, here and there covered with shiny, red, and somewhat elevated spots. Treatment of the most various kind has been employed. *Kali bichrom.* 6 and 3, with simultaneous application of cold water as a gargarism, and nasal suction, as well as cold applications to the throat, soon improved. The discharge soon stopped almost entirely; only occasionally a little blood-streaked mucus appeared; in the throat only a slight sensation of dryness remained, symptoms which gradually disappeared. During the administration of Kal. bichrom. the menstruation ceased, and was delayed even at the next few terms. Simultaneously swollen lips and constipation (Dr. Black, Brit. Jour. of Hom., April, 1857).

---

* In the same manner did *Strophulus confertus* in several children alternate with *Asthma Millari; Acne* and *cutaneous tubercle* with *internal tuberculous irritation; Vitiligo* with *disturbances of the liver.* Finally, after the artificial suppression of a crusty, herpetic eruption of the nose, *Chlorosis* in one case, and an apparent *hypertrophy and enlargement of the heart* in another, both of which evils disappeared upon the use of Calc. carb., under RETURN OF THE ERUPTION.

3. (LXXIII.) *Kali chromicum against Enlarged Tonsils.**

A man, æt. 50, for a long time suffered from swelling of the tonsils and submaxillary glands. At the same time the Eustachian tube was obstructed, and in consequence thereof there existed hardness of hearing. Various remedies had been applied for a good while without result. *Kal. bichromic.* 1, within fourteen days restored the hearing, and within other fourteen days almost completely removed the swelling. The same author employed *Kal. chromic.* with excellent results against torpid swelling of the tonsils, not accompanied by inflammatory symptoms, especially in children of lax, leucophlegmatic constitution, and if loosening of the nasal mucosa and crusts in the nose existed simultaneously (Dr. Drysdale, Brit. Jour. of Hom., 1857).

4. (LXXIV.) *Kali chromicum and bichromicum against Chronic Inflammation of the Nasal Mucosa.*

A woman, æt. 50, who had suffered much from congestion and a sensation of coldness in the head, after an attack of coryza which appeared with the cessation of menstruation, since two years presented the following symptoms: Continual, thick, yellowish discharge from the left nasal opening, which became offensive upon the influence of the open air, and was most copious in the morning. Violent pain in the muscles of the left side of the neck, extending to the head, and called forth and aggravated by blowing the nose. In the nose feeling of soreness extending to the cheeks. Sneezes but rarely; smell undisturbed; general health good, with the exception of some constipation, with a white coating of the tongue. *Kali bichrom.*, now the 6th, now the 3d, or 2d dilution every

* The following notice regarding the physiological action of the Bichromate of Potash is probably of some interest:

"A lean, anæmic man, æt. 30, engaged in a factory with the preparation of Bichromate of Potash, for a few months had had several ulcers on the tonsils and œsophagus, which are covered by an ashy gray crust, and surrounded by a dark-colored, livid, and swollen mucosa. Pulse small, 120; great thirst; tongue dry and red; difficult swallowing and sleeplessness. He stated that all his comrades in the factory were suffering more or less from the same trouble (Lancet, February, 1854; Schmidt's Jahrb., 1851, 82).

other day, and a solution of *Kal. chrom.* (½ grain to ℥j of water) externally, removed the trouble within a fortnight (Dr. Drysdale, Brit. Jour. of Hom., 1857).

### 5. (LXXV.) *Kali chromicum and bichromicum against Chronic Eczema of the Head and Face.*

A healthy servant, æt. 36, for three years suffered from an intensely irritating and burning eruption, which extended over the whole head, almost deprived of all hair, to the eyebrows. The whole surface was red, raw, and discharged a thin matter, here and there drying up into yellow crusts. Rhus, Graph., Mercur., &c., had sufficed temporarily only. *Kal. bichrom.* 2, morning and evening, together with one daily application of a solution of *Kal. bichr. neutr.* (1 grain to 1 ounce of water), soon removed the trouble.

A relapse of it was permanently removed by Kal. chrom. 0, $\frac{1}{20}$th of a grain daily, and the external application mentioned above (Ibidem).

### 6. (LXXVI.) *Coryza Chronica.*

A strong youth, æt. 17; coryza of three years' standing, without interruption, accompanied by heaviness and dulness in the head, nasal voice, and a thin, mucous discharge. *Pulsat.* 2, for fourteen days, did not improve any. *Kal. bichrom.* 4, sixteen doses. Radical cure within eight days (Bolle).

### 7. (LXXVII.) *Catarrh with Hoarseness.*

Kali bichrom., 2d trit., removed a laryngeal catarrh with hoarseness in a singer. Dr. Teller recommends *Kal. bichrom.*, one grain of the 2d trit. in four ounces of water, a teaspoonful from one to two hours, against catarrh, even with feverish conditions of a lighter grade (A. H. Z., 59, 10).

It is not unimportant to know, as we have already mentioned, that *Kal. bichrom.* has also been given advantageously against secondary and tertiary forms of syphilis. Drysdale cured with it syphilitic periostitis and exanthemata, probably of a syphilitic nature (A. H. Z., 55, 14). It seems to be suitable, precisely as is the red precipitate of Mercury, against scrofulo-syphilitic affections.

NOTE.—The CHLORIDE OF POTASSIUM has a characteristic curative action so definite that we will also mention it here. It is the specific remedy against stomacace (always accompanied by a peculiar fetid smell). It is remarkable that both allopaths and homœopaths give it in this disease.

According to the "Homœopathic Times," 1853, No. 188, p. 449, Laurie cured a case of stomacace by *Kal. chlor.*, 1st trit., one grain three times a day, which had developed to such a degree as to cause perforation of the cheek.

And Alfred Vogel says, in his excellent text-book on diseases of children:

"We are so fortunate as to possess *one* remedy against stomacace. By this remark enough is said for its recommendation. It is CHLORIDE OF POTASSIUM." To children less than one year old Vogel gives 20 grains daily; to those less than two years of age, 30 grains; to those less than three years old, 40 grains; and continues, somewhat naively: "Children who have reached the fourth year already bear a drachm of it very well." We know, however, that one needs not give so much of the specific remedy as may be borne.

*Odor fœtidus* from the stomach: Chloride of Potassium, 6, 0 in sugar-water 120, 0, a teaspoonful three hours after eating. (Stanislaus Martin.)

---

## LYCOPODIUM.

### GENERALITIES.

"*Lycopodium* is closely related to Sulphur, which is also contained in the plant from which we obtain the *Lycopodium seeds*." For this reason alone the second designation of Lycopodium, "*Sulphur vegetabilis*" is justified.

By this fact only a series of curative results can be explained, so especially its efficacy in malignant ophthalmia of the new-born* (ophth. neonator.), related to scabies on account of its great contagiousness.

But *Lycopod.* is also a bone-remedy, and suitable in rhachitis (after *Calc. carb.*), if the bones suppurate and become crooked. Further, in chronic skin diseases, incipient caries (similar to Silicea), in ulcers which bleed easily (similar to Mercur.), in suppurating and moistening herpetic eruptions, and suppurating eruptions on the head. Again (besides in ophth. neonat.), in ophthalmia with nocturnal agglutination and watering of the eyes in the open air, sensation of coldness in the eyes in the evening; obscurity of sight, inflammation of the lid-glands, swollen glands of the neck; in gastric symptoms, such as the scrofulous frequently exhibit, especially if chronic constipation and flatulency are connected therewith. In dry coryza with dulness in the head. Against scrofulous coryza, if the discharge is yellowish or greenish. Nose ulcerated and crusty in the inside. (Kal. carb.) Dry cough. Shortness of breathing.

It seems to us as if *Lycopod.* was suitable more to the processes of scrofula, which are not connected with excessive secretion, especially not with a profuse, purulent discharge, for which *Calc. carb*, *Mercur.*, and others are the more appropriate remedies. *Lycopod.* corresponds more to *suppressed* secretions, or to scrofulous processes without discharge, with exsiccation and hardness of the parts (similar to Silicea),† and to Arsenic., which, for example, cures ichthyosis, or to Graphit., which restores the suppressed hæmorrhoidal flow.

One becomes more convinced of this when he considers the curative power of *Lycopod.* in the affections of the plica-polonica-dyscrasia, the principal character of which is sluggishness of the peripheric activities (*e. g.*, of suppressed perspiration), and which offers many points of contact with scrofulosis.

The exanthemata within the confines of the head and face which *Lycopod.* cures, may be *moist*, and suppurate, but lack the thick, fat, and profuse discharge of pus.

---

* Lycopodium 12, internally every two hours, and Lycopod. 6 (four drops in four ounces of water) externally.

† Moreover, Lycopod., precisely like Silicea, is recommended against nocturnal pains in the bones from abuse of Mercury.

*Lycopod.* is especially suitable in hardness of hearing, with discharge of a thin, yellowish liquid from the ear.

In scrofulous tumor albus *Lycopod.* is given in alternation with *Calc. carb.* (and Silicea).

Croup, an eloquent expression of existing scrofulosis, sometimes requires *Lycopod.*, if hoarseness remained, or (in the critical stage) loose cough during the day, and hoarseness and paroxysms of suffocation are present at night; or, as a general thing, if suffocative paroxysms interchange with free intervals.

Finally, we will mention the therapeutic, preventive power of *Lycopod.* in the following affections of the bladder: In the bladder, feeling of heaviness; burning during micturition; constant, and sometimes very violent urging to urinate, with subsequent ischuria; catarrhal inflammation of the bladder; urine turbid, milky, and flocculent; frequent urging, sometimes with the impossibility of passing water, whereby children always hold the lower part of the abdomen, and cry impatiently; in connection therewith a pale and clear urine.

Anuria neonatorum.*

*Lycopodium*, as a general thing, is to be used more in diseases of grown persons than of children. If the theory is correct, according to which scrofula is said to represent a kind of infantile gout, we will think of this remedy, especially when we have to do with children of gouty parents. At this juncture we will again remind the reader of the fact that the rest of the famous gout remedies of our, *i. e.*, the homœopathic therapia, such as *Calc. carb.*, *Silic.*, *Phosph.*, even the preparations of *Iodine*, and especially *Hepar sulph.*, are just as useful and indispensable antiscrofulosa; a decisive momentum, no doubt, in the solution of the question:

Are scrofulous affections related to the arthritic, or not?

---

* It is singular that the allopathic school, which, in its rationality, goes so far as to place this remedy between Ol. ricini and Ol. jec. aselli (see Schœman's Arzneimittellehre, 2 Auflage), also recommends Lycopod. against spasmodic and inflammatory irritation of the urinary organs (dysuria, stranguria, ischuria), as well as against cardialgia. Even the Lycopod. growing on the Antilles is used there internally as a diuretic, and externally against gouty tumors (Altschul. Reallexicon, S. 187).

In contradistinction from *Calc. carb.*, which corresponds more to the pastous form, combined with mental indolence, *Lycopodium* would correspond more to the erethic form.

From Rueckert's "Attempt at utilizing the curative material obtained *ab usu in morbis*," we quote yet the following indications for Lycopodium:

"1. Sensation in the œsophagus as from a hard body, with stitching pains, a feeling of swelling, and morning expectoration of a yellowish, thick mucus, which is firm, almost hard in the centre, and of a greenish-yellow color.

"I have several times had the pleasure of completely curing with *Lycopod.* 30 that disease of the œsophagus, otherwise known to be incurable, which ends with caries of the cervical vertebræ, and which, as the expression of an affection of a very grave nature, we see accompanied by a swollen and irritated mucosa of the throat, varicose vessels, and a herpes-like eruption thereupon, together with small, fleshy excrescences luxuriantly growing and passing into suppuration."

2. Chronic scrofulous eruptions, which always cover themselves freshly with dirty-yellowish, brownish, or greenish crusts, have a nauseating, flat, mouldy, or decaying smell, are partly dry, partly discharging, mostly show a fungus-like formation under the magnifying glass, and predominantly appear upon the hairy parts of the body.

3. The boils preceding panaritium diffusum exhibit the characteristic that they terminate incompletely only, suppurate but little, but become bluish, cease to suppurate, and leave incomplete cicatrices and purple spots.

The boils in and around the axilla, with discharging, crusty, and itching herpetic eruptions upon it, and swelling of the axillary glands. The boils suppurate for a long time, and fresh ones appear continually.

*Lycopodium* is also a coryza remedy.

Present are: *Dryness of the nose*, and acrid secretion, especially, however, an annoying frontal headache (for which *Mercurius* also comes under consideration), with aggravation in the evening, and final blowing out of a lemon-colored mucus (Goullon).

Crusts in the nose; nocturnal agglutination of the nasal openings, with dry coryza (Hahnemann).

Dryness of the choanæ, with offensive nasal secretion, hoarseness, rawness and soreness in the chest; in nocturnal tussis titilans, with a sensation as from sulphur vapors (Kafka).

### CLINIQUE.

#### 1. (LXXVIII.) *Lycopodium against Warts.*

In a scrofulous girl, æt. 6, who was affected with several facial ulcers, corresponding to her constitutional trouble, a considerable number of small, soft, pedicellate warts formed upon the chin over night. When I was shown the child, I remembered having read that Léon Simon successfully employed *Lycopod.* in a similar trouble. I prescribed *Lycopod.* 6, two drops morning and evening, and recommended to moisten the epidermoid formations twice daily with *Lycopod.* tincture, diluted with alcohol. After a few days all the warts disappeared, and the scrofulous ulcers assumed a better appearance.

It is questionable in this case whether the external or internal treatment effected most. Skeptics may attribute a portion of the effect to the influence of the alcohol, yet the action of *Lycopod.* upon scrofulosis and abnormal vegetation has been confirmed in too many cases to admit of any doubt* (Z. f. h. Kl., 4, 21, Verrucæ, Dr. Teller, of Prague).

#### 2. (LXXIX.) *Intertrigo.*

An infant, one year old, suffered from intertrigo. Violent crying when urinating. *Tr. Lycopod.*, in water, internally and externally. Cure within a few days.

#### 3. (LXXX.) *Glandular Swelling.*

Miss S., about 30 years of age, *a true type of the scrofulous habitus*, for more than a year has suffered from glandular

* A. H. Z , 31, 3. Segin took from 20 to 50 drops of the 30th dil. for 5 days. On the third day, papulæ on the legs, stinging like needles. After 8 days, sweat and feeling of soreness between the toes.—Enuresis nocturna.—The latter, as well as the pain in the toes, returned after 14 days. (Never experienced previously.)

swellings. Along the right side of the throat and neck a number of glands, about as large as nutmegs, were observed, which were painless and movable, but very hard. However, a hypertrophical swelling of the submaxillary gland, as big as a man's fist and as hard as cartilage, surpassed all the others. It was firmly fixed, painless, reached far above the level of the jaw, and gave to the scrofulous face a very deforming appearance. Patient had been scrofulous since childhood, but could not remember having had any other diseases, and even presently did not complain of any other trouble except constipation.

Treated without result from January 20th to July 18th with Staphisagria, Sulph., and Calc. carb. (high potencies).

July 18th, August 7th and 22d, and September 9th, three doses of *Lycopodium* (high potency), one to be taken every third day.

Four weeks after the first doses, the effect upon the glandular tumor was perceptible. It began to get movable, could be displaced, and the examining finger could feel a beginning division of the conglomerate. These divisions became more plain from week to week; the swelling separated more and more into single and smaller glandular portions, which severed from another, and thus the hard tumor dissolved, no more medicine being given after the middle of September. At the end of the year the ungainly swelling was entirely removed. The cervical glands were reduced simultaneously.

"I would like to know," Dr. Fielitz concludes, "whether the Mat. Med. of the physiological school possesses remedial powers which cure such an evil more surely and without poisoning by Mercury and Iodine. A cure of this kind by the *vis medicatrix naturæ* alone I have never witnessed in my practice of thirty-six years' standing" (A. H. Z., 52, 14).

---

## MERCURIUS.*

### GENERALITIES.

Experience teaches that the various preparations of this remedy can impress upon and communicate to the whole lymphatic system a peculiar modification, and to the whole economy of the body a tendency similar to the scrofula-dyscrasia. Indeed, John Hunter, Vigaroux, Samuel Cooper, Richerand, Alibert, and others demonstrated that persons who, in consequence of their calling, were exposed to the evil influences of quicksilver, frequently beget scrofulous children. Homœop-

---

* According to A. Lutze, it does not make any difference which preparation of quicksilver is employed, since the symptoms produced by all the various preparations agree. He generally uses, however, *Hydrargyrum oxydatum rubrum* as the purest, and, therefore, most suitable preparation for triturations and potencies. According to Dr. G. Gerson the *red precipitate* is vastly superior in its specific curative action against single forms, especially the scrofulous, to *Merc. solubilis.* He bases his remark upon the relation between scrofulosis and syphilis, and believes that the contagiousness is a characteristic of both. Of the several forms of the scrofula-dyscrasia in which the red precipitate deserves preference, he names:

1. Scrofulous ophthalmia (believing that even its external application is to be considered as a specific and not as a caustic), if the swelling of the conjunctiva is not very considerable, its redness of a bright color, its discharge purulent, and photophobia has not reached its highest degree. Also where troubles from teething were present at the same time.

2. Scrofulous eczematous eruptions which have their principal seat at the flexor-planes of the extremities, especially near the joints and at the musculi glutæi, and are characterized by the severity of the pains. The discharged pus is contagious. The healing up starts at the centre of the plaques.

3. Scrofulous bubo with acute inflammatory irritation and tendency to suppuration. The pains quickly ameliorate, and where resorption does not take place, suppuration appears soon, and is of benign nature, without any turbid ulcers developing at the opened spot.

4. A peculiar form of scrofulous ulcers among girls and boys from 4 to 10 years of age, which entirely simulates the character of syphilis. Among boys the ulcers appeared at the anterior portion of the penis, on the præputium and scrotum; among girls at the labia and urethral orifice, and even at the perineum. They lacked the hardness of the subcutaneous cellular tissue. Characteristic, is their painfulness and the sympathetic irritation and swelling of the inguinal glands.

5. Scrofulous superficial ulcers developing from large, doughy tumors at the neck and thorax.

athy has good reason to hold on to this experience without, however, overrating this source of scrofulosis. Because we are indebted to it for a series of genuine curative results, which furnish at the same time a brilliant testimony of the truth of our therapeutic principle, "Similia similibus curantur."

The physiological effect of *Mercury* upon the salivary glands is most remarkable and known. Dieterich (Mercurial Krankheiten, Leipzig, 1837), above all, counts the "*hypertrophy of the glands*," *i. e.*, the enlargement of the *inguinal*, *axillary*, *mesenterical* glands, of the *parotis*, the *pancreas*, and even the *testes* and *liver*, among his forms of mercurial dyscrasia. Increase of the glandular secretion is almost always connected therewith. *Mercury*, hence, has been the first refuge in all glandular diseases, and, as a general thing, is still considered as one of the principal remedies in scrofulosis (glandular diseases). But as there can be no exclusive panacea against diseases of single systems or organs, the use of *Mercury* also has been carried too far, and its administration in diseases of the glands ought to be restricted without any doubt (Dr. Reil, N. Z. f. h. Kl., 1, 9).

As regards its influence upon the osseous system, *Mercurius* is closely related to Silicea, and in fact is utterly indispensable in most of the scrofulous processes by virtue of its property as a suppuration remedy. We mention, moreover, of the mercurial effects pertaining here: "inflammatory, especially nocturnal pains in the bones; crookedness and great fragility of the bones. Eruptions resembling scabies florida, or dry, rash-like, easily bleeding, itch. Inflammatory swelling of the glands; suppurations of every kind; swelling of the head, or eruptions upon it; ophthalmia, especially if the lids are red and swollen; tearing and itching pains in the ears; purulent or bloody discharge; hardness of hearing with bellowing and roaring in the ears; also in otitis interna acuta with violent nocturnal pains and suppuration (Trinks); inflammation and swelling of the nose, especially of its tip; stomacace; angina with swelling of the tonsils and copious flow of saliva;" (Angina tonsillarum ulcerosa—Goullon).

For scrofulosis erethica et florida, inflammation of the glands with phlegmonous redness, swelling and pains aggravating in the evening, *Mercur.* is especially suitable. Further in blepharoadenitis of scrofulous persons (here surpassed or complemented only by Silic.). Ulceration of the cornea and photophobia.

Though not always connected with scrofulosis, angina uvularis (elongated and swollen uvula) presents a perspicuous proof of the therapeutic action of *Mercury.* Dr. Bolle (Aachen) has been first in pointing out that such an inflammation, even if it has already become chronic, gives way amazingly quickly to the influence of sublimate.*

Trinks, moreover recommends *Mercurius* against atrophia meseraica, pot-bellies of children who mostly have been brought up by hand, with diarrhœa and fever from teething. Hartmann's recommendation in mastitis, in which Mercury is said to hasten suppuration, confirms the analogy between this remedy and Silic. mentioned by us. Both remedies resemble each other also in their curative power against coxalgia (claudicatio spontanea).

Again, the greatly experienced Trinks calls *Merc.* (sol.) one of the most efficacious remedies against coryza with copious discharge of a corroding (mucous—Baer) liquid, and finally against the inflammatory stage of panaritium. Here it ameliorates the pain, hastens the formation of pus, and again, unquestionably, shows its therapeutic relation to Silicea. But why do we administer Silic. in one case, and *Mercurius* in the other? What is the essential difference between remedies apparently agreeing so much?

## SILICEA.

Bone-remedy.

Aggravation at the time of the new moon and full moon; pains on changes of weather.

Indurations (scirrhous).

Herpetic eruptions.

Beginning suppuration, or defective suppressed suppuration.

Suppressed sweat of the feet.

---

* A few grains of a lower trituration mixed with four ounces of distilled water, and used as a gargarism, suffice.

Yellow, crippled, and brittle finger-nails.
CONSTIPATION.

### MERCURIUS.

Gland-remedy.
Appearance of the symptoms at night (in the warm bed).
Established suppuration.
Easily bleeding ulcers.
Bloody discharge from the ear.
Bloody, blood-streaked, and bloody-mucous diarrhœa.
LOOSENESS OF THE BOWELS.

*Mercurius* more resembles *Calc. carb.*, *Caustic.*, *Phosph.*, and *Acid nitr.* *Silicea*, on the contrary, finds its best analogue in *Arsenic* (besides in *Graphit.* and *Lycopod.*), and in common with it has "*vomiting every time after drinking.*" The antagonism existing between *Silic.* and *Mercur.*, notwithstanding all similarity, already follows from the fact that *Silicea* cures ulcers which owe their origin to abuse of *Mercury.*

### CLINIQUE.

### MERCURIUS SOLUBILIS.

#### 1. (LXXXI.) *Ophthalmia Scrofulosa.*

Mercur. sol. Hahn. 2, one grain morning and evening, within five weeks cured a genuine scrofulous ophthalmia of three months' standing. Flow of acrid tears corroding the cheeks. Lids swollen ; a pustular eruption upon them and the cheeks ; dried-up pus on the ciliæ. Whitish-gray spots have formed upon the cornea of both eyes. Photophobia. The child lies upon its face continually. Nose and lips swollen ; a copious, green, thick, and acrid mucus, which makes the nasal openings and upper lip sore, flows out of the former. The profuse nasal discharge requires constant wiping. The outer surface of the hand and the outer side of the lower part of the forearm, with which the child wipes off the acrid nasal discharge, are corroded by it. The parotid glands are swollen; the child is very ill-humored and impatient, and cries almost constantly.

Several remedies, also *Arsenic* (high and low), had remained without any effect.

2. (LXXXII.) *Offensive Otorrhœa with Polypous Formations, Chronic Inflammation of the Membrana Tympani, and Hardness of Hearing.**

After the measles (in the sixth year), otorrhœa. The smell of the discharge so offensive that nobody could remain near the patient, and its quantity so great that clothing and pillows were really wet with it.

The right meatus closed by a soft polypus. Mucosa of the meatus red, loosened, sore, and tender. Hearing distance on the right side = 0.

To be taken, two grains of Merc. sol. H. 3 in the evening. (Externally, frequent injections of tepid water, and powdering of the meatus with one grain of Merc. sol. H.)

The offensive smell of the discharge, as well as the discharge itself, decreased rapidly, and the polypus became detached after using the remedy for six days. At the inmost and posterior portion of the meatus (at this spot polypi of the meatus almost always originate) only a trace was to be seen of the spot where the polypus was inserted, but the membrana tympani presented a dark-red, granular (frog's-spawn-like), convex surface, which proved itself very tender on touch with the probe.

Distance of hearing, two inches.

Upon the continued internal use of Merc. sol. H., two grains every other evening, and daily injections of tepid water, the otorrhœa entirely ceased within four weeks, the granulations upon the membrana tympani and meatus likewise disappeared, the hearing distance increased to 8″, the roaring in the ear passed away, but the sound of the tuning-fork was still heard stronger on the right (?) side.

3. (LXXXIII.) *Stomacace.*

One dose of Mercur. sol. H. 2, gr. j, removed aphthæ, bad

* Beitraege zur Erkenntniss u. Behandlung einiger Ohrenkrankheiten. Von Dr. Rentsch, in Potsdam, XXXVIII, 5.

breath, swelling of the glands, diarrhœa, and fever-heat in the evening in a child.

4. (LXXXIV.) *Angina tonsillaris.*

In the same manner a violent case of angina tonsillaris, with intense redness, great swelling of the left tonsil, nasal voice, a swelling below the left lower jaw of the size of a hen's-egg, and painful high fever, in a patient æt. 20, gave way without any unpleasant consequences and subsequent suppuration within three days, upon two doses of *Mercur. sol.* 4, gr. ij (Hygea, 15, 4).

The above reminds us of Dr. Goetze's remark, who, while reporting several handsome cures by *Mercury*, says: "*Merc. sol. Hahn.* 3 is specific in most cases of angina with swelling of the *tonsils* or *submaxillary glands*, especially in that form of angina in which *caseous* exudations are observed at an early hour upon the inflamed portions of the mucosa, and which must be designated as *croupous*, though not as truly diphtheritic."

5. (LXXXV.) *Periostitis.*

In a feeble child, five years old, who got sick under febrile symptoms, and had pains in one of its lower legs, a swelling developed at that locality, and especially at the tibial region, which was very sensitive on the slightest touch even.

Upon the administration of *Merc. sol. H.* 3, a dose from two to three hours, with simultaneous wrapping up of the leg in raw cotton, the intensity of the violent fever, as well as the local phenomena, decreased as early as within a few days, and I succeeded in curing the intense periostitis within the course of one week without any suppuration following (Dr. Goetze, of Itzehoe, A. H. Z., 79, 12).

6. (LXXXVI.) *Eczema.*

Paul Dubois, who saturated the whole body with large doses of *Mercury* for the purpose of curing a case of peritonitis puerperalis, frequently produced thereby eczemata. Dr. Banks, of New York, remembered this fact and removed with Merc. sol. (1 : 10), five grains of the first trituration, given from four to five times daily, an eczema that had been treated without success for four years. The case occurred in a tall weakly girl, æt. 9½, with delicate skin, blue eyes, and flaxen hair. The skull was completely covered with a thin yellowish crust, which had burst on many places and discharged a pale, straw-colored, and viscid liquid. The hair was matted together, and came out. Behind the ear a raw, cherry-red, secreting surface. This spot was completely surrounded by small vesicles of different stages of development. There were similar spots on the face, neck, and shoulders.

The disease had begun with a circular, eczematous eruption at the occiput (*Arsenic*, *Hep. sulph.*, *Sulph.*, *Rhus*, &c.). Washing with alkalies and acids only aggravated.

After using *Mercur. sol.* for a few days in the manner mentioned there was decided improvement. In three weeks almost a complete cure. But two doses daily. In eight weeks a complete cure and luxuriant growth of the hair.

Dr. Banks reports having cured two other similar cases of eczema with the same success by *Mercury* (North Americ. Journ., May, 1857).

---

## NATRUM.

### *A.*—NATRUM MURIATICUM.

#### GENERALITIES.

Chronic skin diseases; urticarious and miliary eruptions. Boils, pustules, and eruption on the face, especially at the corners of the mouth. Profuse night-sweats. Watering of the eyes (in the open air). Snapping of the eyelids; obscurity of sight. Roaring in the ears. Hardness of hearing. Purulent discharge from the ears. Swelling of the submaxillary glands, lips, and cervical glands. Strumatous glandular swellings (the same as in scrofulous persons). Easy bleeding of the gums. Looseness of the teeth. Hard stool alternating with diarrhœa. *Hoarseness. Pain in the larynx and trachea.*

Dyspnœa ; purulent expectoration at coughing (tuberculosis). Can any one find any more pregnant symptoms of scrofulosis than in these characteristic drug-effects of the common Chloride of Sodium? For this reason we do not doubt for a moment the reports of French physicians who observed that sea-salt, solved in water, proved itself efficacious against scrofulous ulcers upon the cornea with photophobia.*

Otherwise, the clinical use that has thus far been made of *Natrum muriaticum* in scrofulous troubles, is proportionally little. In consideration of the great pathogenetic range of the remedy, its principal character, "*Weariness* and *weakness*" ought to be kept in view.

*Natrum muriaticum* (with the exception of Kali) mostly resembles *Lycopodium* probably, which shows, however, more direct relations to scrofulosis.

And, now, a few more especial indications:

*Natr. mur.* is indicated in *fluent* coryza, alternating with *dry* coryza which is accompanied by hoarseness, a scratching and digging sensation in the trachea, or tussis titilans, in which, however, the irritation producing the cough starts at the epigastrium (status gastricus). Entire absence of taste and smell. Finally, in case of continuous watering of the eyes on account of obstruction of the canalis lachrymalis.†

Lastly, we will quote yet a few of the exceedingly practical remarks from Rueckert's "attempt at utilizing the curative material obtained *ab usu in morbis.*"

The pure kitchen salt is one of the most active antipsoric remedies.

v. Grauvogl mentions it as one of the drugs corresponding to the *hydrogenoid* constitution.

The totality of its action is expressed in its decided influence upon vegetative life.

The lymphatic and nervous systems are principally affected

---

* The observation of Busch that eyes which pain intensely when they are washed with river-water, can be kept open for a longer time without pain in sea-water, and that even distilled water irritates the eyes, while that containing a small portion of salt, does not do so, is instructive.

† There is also a kind of coryza accompanied by an increase of smell. This is cured by Phosphorus (Trinks). In case of a complication with hoarseness and bronchial catarrh.

by *Natr. mur.*, and this already shows its especial adaptation to chronic diseases.

The intermitting character of the trouble still more points to *Natr. mur.*, which, otherwise, can easily be confounded with *Lycopodium.* The latter circumstance argues in favor of its antiscrofulous action. Under certain conditions *Natr. mur.* seems to be especially suitable in ophthalmia scrofulosa. One of these conditions is the secretion of acrid tears, corroding nose and upper lip. Obstruction of the canalis lacrymalis. Again: turbid look of the eyes; suppuration of the cornea. Watering of the eyes, aggravated in the open air. Photophobia with stitching pains in the eyes. Eruptions at the mouth, lips, *corners of the mouth;* pustules; crusts; ulcers (similar to *Graphit.* and *Causticum*).

Scrofulous persons are frequently afflicted with constipation, and in this condition *Natr. mur.* is a remedy that has removed such obstructions of the most stubborn kind. Such momenta must strictly be taken in consideration, if we wish to give to *Natr. mur.* the preference over the many antiscrofulous remedies with more numerous indications, and do not want to regret our choice.*

## *B.*—NATRUM CARBONICUM.

### CLINIQUE.

#### 1. (LXXXVII.) *Coryza Chronica.*

A young girl, æt. 16, of lymphatic constitution, pale face, rings around the eyes, delaying and feeble menstruation, for years suffers from coryza, accompanied by discharge of a thick and copious mucus during the day, and obstruction of the nose at night. Her voice has assumed a very disagreeable, nasal sound. Since the middle lobe of the thyroid gland was swollen, a dosis of Spongia 3, was given morning and evening. But her condition remained the same three weeks afterwards. Now, after *Natr. carbon*, $\frac{6}{5}$ had been given in the same man-

* If we wish to use *Natr. mur.*, in the form of baths, it is done by mixing brine with river-water (equal parts), or by adding one pound of common salt and one pound of sea salt to common warm water.

ner for four weeks, the secretion of mucus has nearly become normal; the gland, still somewhat swollen, had become softer, less resistant, and four weeks afterwards both troubles were completely removed.

### 2. (LXXXVIII.) *Coryza Chronica.*

A lady, æt. 40, who supported herself by singing, took cold in the concert room, and her skin did not perspire since, on the contrary remained entirely dry. What annoyed her most was a chronic coryza with abundant discharge and an unpleasant effect upon her voice.

*Sulphur* aggravated. Sach. lact. to wait for the action of the remedy. No result. *Natrum carbon.* cured the coryza and restored the normal activity of the skin (Hirsch of Prague, A. H. Z.).

---

## PHOSPHORUS.

### GENERALITIES.

For the very reason that *Phosph.* frequently complements and completes the curative action of *Silicea*, *e. g.*, in cases of mastitis and its terminations, we may infer its antiscrofulous character. Like Silicea it is a bone-remedy, but still more a lung-remedy. However, its antiscrofulous character shows itself more distinctly in croup, and just in the most dangerous forms of genuine croup, which rightfully is counted among the characteristic expressions of the scrofula-dyscrasia. Acting, as it does (even according to the views of the old school), as an irritant upon depressed nerve-force, it has done wonders even in the last stage of croup, and at this point mention may be made of the physiological action of *Phosphorus:* "Pulse scarcely perceptible; cold, clammy sweat; chronic hoarseness; burning in the larynx." Moreover, its curative action in chronic diarrhœa, by which scrofulous children are afflicted in the period of dentition and afterwards, in which only *Calc. carb.*, *Calc. acetica*, and *Arsen.* contend with it for supremacy, is well known.

Otherwise, as regards the curative action of *Phosph.* in the special forms of scrofula, its use must be called limited. Aside from its effect upon croup in the last stage with rattling respiration in the upper portion of the chest and trachea (Goullon, Sr.), and in diseases of the bones, such as caries, scrofulosa with hectic fever, and exostoses (Trinks, Knorre), it plays an important part in ozæna narium scrofulosa (Strecker). We could ask the question, moreover, whether the well-known action of *Phosph.* to produce necrosis of the maxillæ has not been taken advantage of in homœopathy. We believe that we can answer in the affirmative, since we possess in *Phosph.* a valuable remedy against toothache of carious teeth (which form, so to say, a part of the jaw). *Phosph.* corresponds to caries *sicca* (*Mercur.* to caries *humida*). Both kinds of toothache undoubtedly count among the annoying privileges of scrofulous individuals.

## CLINIQUE.

### 1. (LXXXIX.) *Croup.*

The daughter of teacher P., five years of age, was attacked by croup in the night from the 20th to the 21st of March. The family physician, who had been called immediately, prescribed an emetic of Tart. stibiat. and Radix ipecac., which produced repeated vomiting, but no change in the course of the disease. On the next day, after a second physician had been called in, leeches were applied to the throat, and calomel was given internally, but the disease rose to its highest degree in spite of this treatment continued up to the third day. In the evening of that day, after the physicians in attendance had pronounced the prognosis to be most unfavorable, the distressed father requested Dr. Vehsemeyer to take charge of the child.

The latter found the little patient lying in bed, purple in the face, covered with cold sweat, looking about in agony, and periodically boring her head backward into the pillow; respiring with a highly raised chest and stretched neck; then again hastily rising in the greatest distress, grasping herself at the throat and pulling her hair. Respiration wheezy and whistling; voice whispering; speaks by hastily thrusting out single words; cough soundless. Larynx and trachea painful upon touch; pulse small, irregular, and not countable on account of its frequency.

During the night five grains of the 2d trit. of Hepar sulph. and Spongia,* every hour in alternation, were given to the child, and sponges, dipped in hot water, laid upon its throat. There was not the slightest improvement on the next morning, the fourth day of the sickness. Now two drops of the undiluted *Spiritus Phosphori*, in sugar-water, were given every hour, but already after a few hours the child was not able any more to swallow. I found her apathetic, with her lower jaw hanging down, her eyes deeply sunken and half closed, only now and then making efforts of breathing; face and hands bloated, purple, cool, the whole body covered with cold sweat. Cough set in, but very seldom, in single, soundless thrusts; (abdominal) respiration irregular, voice entirely gone. The unfortunate parents stood, loudly crying, at the bedside of their darling, and I had to confess to myself that there was no hope in this case. At that instant the thought flashed through Dr. Vehsemeyer's mind to try externally what could not be administered any longer internally. Phosph., gr. 2, with Ol. amygdal. dulc. ℥ß, was prescribed. This was to be rubbed in every ten minutes upon throat and chest, and the latter to be covered with flannel. After this treatment had been continued for 1½ hours, the child showed signs of returning life by reaching at her throat, and making the motion of rubbing in a distressed and imploring manner. Now the inunctions were repeated at longer intervals (from 1¼ to 1½ hours). The cough, still soundless though, returned.† During the night the child began to swallow again, and forthwith *Spirit. Phosph.* was resumed in the dose mentioned above. On the morning of the fifth day, the little patient had improved so far that the most dangerous symptoms were removed, and her condition resembled that in which Dr. Vehse-

* Vehsemeyer calls these "*his usual croup remedies*," and at the beginning of the disease they seem to be sufficient, indeed, and render leeches, Spanish flies, and especially emetics superfluous.

† Also C. A. Tietze calls the entire disappearance of cough in croup "*an ominous symptom.*"

meyer had found her on his first visit. In the course of the day, the cough became more frequent, and though remaining dry, reassumed the usual croup-sound; respiration became more even, yet remained accelerated and whistling (rhonchus sibilans), and was still predominantly abdominal, the chest raising but little, and the intercostal spaces not expanding any. Yet the paroxysms of distress, less frequent though, returned, during which the child begged for the inunctions. Thus intermissions of shorter or longer duration set in. The pulse remained still small and exceedingly frequent (135); the urine showed a white sediment; the expression of the face was less distressed, except during the real paroxysms. *Phosph.* was continued, externally and internally, in smaller doses, and given less frequently (2d dil., 3 drops). In the course of the sixth day, the cough finally assumed the catarrhal sound, and brought up several coherent, firm pieces of mucus, with evident relief to the patient, respiration began to rattle (mucous rattling), the pulse became stronger and less frequent, the skin warm and moist with perspiration; the voice, however, was still without any sound.

For the following six days Hep. sulph. c. 2 was given, at first frequently, afterwards in rare doses. During this time the cough became more and more loose, large pieces of coherent mucus (no real membranes) were thrown up, respiration became more and more free and deeper, the appetite returned, only the voice of the child remained without sound; and not before six weeks afterwards, when the child had already recovered and left her bed for some time, did the voice, still hoarse though, assume a louder sound, which, two years later even, was muffled, and deprived of its metallic tone.*

### 2. (XC.) *Croup.*

A. K., son of Prof. K., a weakly, scrofulous boy, ten years old, one morning, when just at the eve of taking his breakfast, was suddenly seized by a violent and distressing sen-

* Let it be mentioned here that Dr. Vehsemeyer published this certainly highly instructive cure on account of Dr. Elb's remark, "*that Phos. was not exerting any curative action in genuine croup*" (S.; A. H. Z., 51, 8).

sation of suffocation and cough, with croupous sound. As soon as his mother heard this sound, too well known to her only, she immediately applied for help. Half an hour later Dr. V. found the boy with all the phenomena of croup, and an allopathic physician already engaged with the application of leeches, three of which were already drawing. Notwithstanding the immediate removal of the leeches, it was no easy matter to arrest the bleeding, which reappeared at every fresh outbreak of cough. For this reason no application of warm water, highly valued by Dr. V., could be made.

He gave patient Hep. sulph. calc. and Spongia, without, however, removing by this treatment, which was continued for twelve hours, the existing danger; for, although decided intermissions set in, the cough nevertheless retained its rough, barking sound, the respiration remained sawing, and the paroxysms of distress, less frequent though, were more violent, so that Dr. V. concluded to give four drops of the 1st dil. of *Spirit. Phosphori* every hour, by means of which he succeeded, after the disease had lasted eighteen hours, in bringing about a favorable crisis, which, in this instance, was hastened by the administration of Tart. stib. 2. The latter remedy was indicated by an uncommonly strong, full, and widely diffused mucous rattling (A. H. Z., 51, 9).

### 3. (XCI.) *Bronchitis Capillaris.*

The following case proves the direction in which *Phosph.* develops its curative action, as well as the connection (metaschematismus), recently doubted by authors of name, between the cutaneous organ and inflammatory processes in the interior of the body.

A child, six months old, for three months suffered from eczema, producing discharging crusts, which occupied forehead and cheeks; two older children of the same family had been scrofulous. The eczema now began to dry up suddenly; the mother of the child denying, however, of having applied any external remedy. The child coughed, and the cough increased in the ratio in which the eczema diminished; hoarseness; expectoration of glassy mucus; the cough, appearing in paroxysms, tormented the child day and night. Hepar sulph.

without result. On the second day fever, accelerated respiration and pulse. Child lies in bed with a distressed expression on the face; mucous rattling over both lungs.

Tart. emet. 1 in solution, a teaspoonful every hour.

In the following night the child is in a very critical condition. Pulse small, quick, and intermitting; face purple; heat over the whole body; abdominal respiration; crackling, with mucous rattling. In this case of bronchitis capillaris, connected with the greatest danger of life, Dr. Schleicher now administered *Phosph.* 1 in water, a teaspoonful every half hour.

As early as after one hour the child respired more freely, and expectorated; expression on face more quiet and content. 6 A.M., quiet sleep.

Pulse energetic again; temperature of the skin moderate; respiration free. *Phosph.* every three hours. Three days afterwards the affection was completely cured; but at the same time *the eczema began to develop again*, and a week later was at its height.

One dose of *Sulph.* 3, every morning, cured the eruption within three weeks, without any subsequent affection of the lungs, or relapse (A. H. Z., 55, 2).

### 4. (XCII.) *Scarlatina Scrofulosa.*

In the meeting of the homœopathic physicians of Saxony, at Dresden, August 30th, 1857, Hirschel reported a case of scarlatina scrofulosa, with convulsions, in which, after the administration of *Zinc. met.* 1, sopor and collapse of the vital forces, stertorous respiration, involuntary discharge of urine and fæces appeared, and in which considerable improvement set in on the same day after *Phos.* 2. The exanthema did not break out until the day following, so that the good result cannot be attributed to it, but to *Phosphorus* (A. H. Z., 55, 4).

### 5. (XCIII.) *Phthisis Incipiens.*

There have been many discussions on the question, whether tuberculosis and scrofulosis are one and the same dyscrasia. Since there are remedies which are able to arrest the tuberculous process, as well as the scrofulous, we are undoubtedly compelled, to a certain extent, to consider both identical. Among these remedies, especially, *Phosphor.* belongs, and the following case will probably suffice as illustrative of this view:

A landed proprietor of Krajoda, thirty some years of age, slenderly built, brunette, was declared to be consumpted by Drs. Sigmund and Oppolzer. Patient has had many chancres, and frequently gonorrhœa.

Great weakness of all functions; *dry, short cough;* pain in the chest; flabbiness of the muscles; great nervous irritability; want of appetite. Discharge of a mucous liquid from the urethra. Severe pain in the lower part of the back, and irregularity of the bowels.

Six doses of *Phosph.* 30, a dose of six pellets every eighth day, completely cured the patient, who now feels entirely strong and healthy again.

### 6. (XCIV.) *Bronchitis.*

(My own observation.)

O. S., ten weeks old, could be nursed only the first week. Since that time he lives on cows' milk diluted with water (2:1), and some salep mixed with it, without gaining in flesh, however. *On the contrary, the little face frequently looks miserably and full of wrinkles, like the face of a little old man. From the beginning of his life he suffered much from flatulency,* cried much, and drew up his legs similar to one who has severe pain in the bowels. He but very rarely slept quietly, and several hours at a time, and when he drinks, does it so greedily, that he frequently chokes; and then he cries again, until he falls into a sleep, which, however, is but short, and often interrupted.

In the third week he was attacked by a cough, which disappeared and reappeared in alternation. At present it is loose, but the poor little fellow has such a rattling on the chest, as makes one feel always as if he should help him clear the throat.

His stool is not watery, and looks yellow. He has an evacuation, probably, four times within twenty-four hours.

*Phosph.* 30, five pellets every morning. Eight days afterwards: "Your powders have had a very good effect, especially on the stool. He usually has a stool now of firm consistency twice within twenty-four hours. Since about eight days we all see that he improves very satisfactorily, he is much fleshier, and feels a good deal better."

This child, whose mother is exceedingly scrofulous, grew up to be a stout boy, but had a permanent disposition to cough. He is affected by that chronic swelling of the tonsils, which apparently characterizes a dyscrasia, standing midway between scrofulosis and tuberculosis (A. H. Z., 74, 8).

Moleschott (Kreislauf des Lebens, S. 44), as well as G. Rose and Bromeis, are of the opinion that Phosph. acid (and Fluor), is introduced into our blood and bones by the consumption of barley. For this reason Kafka orders barley, either roasted as coffee, or broken up and put into soup, or boiled with milk, to pap for children, in whom the formation of bone goes on slowly. On using this article of diet he observed the repair of matter in general, and, above all, the formation of the bony substance to go on more rapidly (see Die Anæmie oder Blutblaesse, Eine pathol. and therapeut. Studie, A. H. Z., 59, 21).

L. C., "a chronic, *dry, and short cough*, with vague stitches *deeply in the breast*, which, though not continuous, hinder respiration, and increase on deep respiration," is mentioned among the symptoms of an impending or freshly developing tuberculous localization.

Since Cod-liver oil (especially the brown), aside from Iodine, contains *Phosph.* (0,0114 in 100,000), a fact of essential importance, we are probably justified in supposing that this old remedy has frequently owed its results to this circumstance. It was applied then, we may say, in cases which were appropriate for small homœopathic doses of *Phosphorus*.

---

## PETROLEUM.

### GENERALITIES.

*Petroleum* is an important remedy in scrofulous diseases of the ear. When the Eustachian tube participates in the coryza which occasions the most various noises, such as bellowing, roaring, crackling in the ears, we likewise think of *Petr.* Kafka gives *Petrol.* in coryza with hoarseness and obstruction of the choanæ, accumulation in the œsophagus, with pressing, tickling, and roaring; in tussis titilans nocturna, with dryness of the trachea.

Besides, *Petrol.* has cured facial hemiplegia (of scrofulous children). I will not omit the remark, however, that my observations in two cases gave negative results.

## RHUS TOXICODENDRON.

### GENERALITIES.

Dr. Gentzke says of *Rhus:* Its beneficial action in the first stage of coxarthrocace, which colleague Ressig of Berlin has tested in several cases, seems to confirm itself. (This remark is preceded by the report of a cure of coxarthrocace by *Rhus:* 6.) Meyer praises *Rhus* against eczema (besides Sulphur).

### CLINIQUE.

#### 1. (XCV.) *Luxatio Spontanea.*

Mary H., æt. 6, who formerly has suffered from glandular swellings at the neck, which suppurated, assumed a dragging gait in walking, and had pain in the hip-joint, which was increased by pressure upon the large trochanter. Violent pains set in, however, if upon fixing the pelvis, some one with a jerk pressed the femoral head into the acetabulum, one of the surest diagnostic signs of this disease. There could be observed as yet no elongation of the leg and flattening of the glutæi muscles.

The trouble had already existed for from three to four weeks with amelioration alternating with aggravation, the latter being wont to set in amid the appearance of febrile symptoms and with drawing pains in the leg. Forbidding all motions I gave *Rhus* 6 every evening, afterwards less often. The result was favorable. Six weeks later the child could stand upon the leg without pain, and the dragging gait had entirely disappeared.

### 2. (XCVI.) *Ophthalmia Scrofulosa.*

Mary S., æt. 10, has already suffered from scrofulous ophthalmia for four years. Swelling and redness of the conjunctiva with injected vessels and swelling of the sclerotica at the outer edge of the cornea. Spots on the cornea and opacity of the same; photophobia; bloatedness of the face, especially around the nose, the skin of which appears rough; glandular suppuration behind the right ear; watery discharge from the nose.

Sulph., Calcar., and Bellad., without result.

Three doses of *Rhus* 3, two drops as a dose, once a day, for the first few days produced aggravation, and by the secondary action of the remedy, great improvement.

Since, fourteen days later, the improvement seemed to have come to a halt, I gave a few more drops of Rhus 18, and again with the most favorable result; complete cure (Erfahrungen aus der Praxis, Haustein XXXIX, 10).

Note.—Eruptions on the head dependent upon scrofula are cured by Rhus, if a greenish-yellow liquid oozes out, which dries up into yellow, thick crusts, and if the trouble is at the same time of an herpetic nature, itches violently at night, and causes the hair to come out. Other characteristic effects of the remedy are: wet tinea, herpes upon the hairy scalp, ophthalmia; œdematous swelling of the entire eye and its surroundings. Inflammatory swelling of the parotis. For this reason Rhus has clinically proved its efficacy in scrofulous ophthalmia; in parotitis after scarlatina, and in induration of the parotis.

## SILICEA.

### GENERALITIES.

"Silicea est le grand médicament de la scrofule."—Jousset.

The primary effects of *Silicea* manifest themselves in the cerebro-spinal system and the *vegetation of the bones.* As a curative remedy it is especially useful against paralysis in the most extended sense, hence, in chronic weakness of the higher nerve-apparatus, generally; in suppressed capacity of feeling and motion, *suppressed* secretions, especial peripheric, hence, for the same reason in *processes of suppuration* thwarted by the former. Moreover, it is one of the principal remedies in pseudo erysipelas, boils, carbuncles, panaritia, caries, swellings of the bones, and hard tumors.

Dr. Noack, Jr., recommends *Silic.* in scrofulous cutaneous eruptions, if they occupy more the hairy parts (cuir chevelu), and against such as we observe at the tip of the nose.*

He says, in his excellent essay on "*Silicea in processes of suppuration*" (L'Art Médical, March, 1865), "Massive and repeated doses are indicated, if we have to do with (scrofulous) glandular swellings without suppuration. But where there is actually suppuration, or even a tendency thereto only, high dilutions (30th) help." In chronic cases we are in the habit of giving Silicea once a day (and even less often) in subacute cases, morning and evening, and in acute cases from two to three hours.

As regards the power of *Silic.* to restore suppressed sweat of the feet (which, no doubt, sometimes may become a vital point), the A. H. Z., 73, 10, contains five examples, sufficiently supported by the name of Gallivardin, in which mention is made also of the apparent contradiction that, *vice versâ*, *Silicea* cures morbidly increased sweat of the feet in a similar manner as Calc. carb. in a homœopathic dose can cure strumata; and again, that overfeeding with carbonate of lime produces such.†

Icy coldness of the feet, ephidrosis, offensive sweat of the feet (Hartmann), affections of the chest and stomach after suppression of sweat of the feet (Nūnez), all call for *Silicea.* Jousset says of *Silicea:* "It corresponds to pustulous eruptions

---

* Schwarze had given *Graphit.*, with the best result, to a man æt. 23, whose face was covered with eczema, and showed a number of fissures and sores. However, eyelids and mouth had not yet healed. Two doses of *Silicea* (one drop of *Silic.* 30 pro dosi), cured within three weeks.

† Among other remedies which cure abnormal sweat of the extremities, yet are able to restore normal perspiration that has been suppressed, Dr. Gallivardin names: Lycopod., Kali carb., Calc. carb., Sepia, Ammon. carb, and Baryta carb., according to the individuality of the case.

on the head and extremities, and to suppuration of the lymphatic glands. Among its symptoms it has swelling of the abdomen and nose and dry coryza (le coryza épais).*

Otorrhœa, with or without caries; leucorrhœa, chronic diarrhœa. Ophthalmia with ulceration of the cornea; torpid abscesses; caries of the phalanges, the clavicula, and long bones; tumor albus; phthisis with purulent expectoration.

*Suppression of bones and soft tissues point to* SILICEA.

### CLINIQUE.

#### 1. (XCVII.) *Caries of the Right Metatarsal Bones,*

In Franzisca F., æt. 13, who formerly suffered from swollen submaxillary glands. One year ago affected by nettle-rash, which healed spontaneously.

The back of the foot swollen and reddened; two openings upon it at a distance of one inch from each other,—the upper about as large as a good-sized pea, the lower somewhat smaller, which discharges a good deal of greenish pus. At the edges of the openings, in form of a wall, growth of wild flesh. Especially at night she complains of tearing pain in the whole right foot. Besides tearing and stitches in the forehead, noise as from bell-ringing in the ears; vomiting of food.

Mezereum $2^x$, a drop morning and evening, had improved considerably; after it had been taken for six weeks a piece of bone, half a line thick, and about half an inch long, had become detached; the other concomitant symptoms had not improved any. *Iodium* removed the vomiting of food and the other nervous symptoms, but I could not observe any effect from it upon the disease of the bone.

Mercur. improved after four weeks. But the disease of the bone was cured entirely only *after Silicea, one grain of the 3d trituration, had been given for three weeks* (Erfahrungen durch die Praxis vom Wundarzt Haustein zu Gottesgab, Böhmen).

---

* In simultaneous chronic tonsillitis and painless swelling of the submaxillary glands (Kafka).

### 2. (XCVIII.) *Spondylarthrocace.*

Dr. Kämpfer (A. H. Z., 24, 9) cured a case of spondylarthrocace with *Silic.* $\frac{3}{30}$. Afterwards *Calc. carb.* $\frac{3}{30}$.

"I several times observed scrofulous caries of long duration in children to heal within a short time after a few doses of *Silic.* 30, a few pellets at the time (though larger doses were required in other cases)."

### 3. (XCIX.) *Abscess of the Upper Leg.*

In a boy, about two years old, a large inflammatory swelling developed at the right upper leg. A surgeon had ordered the application of some herbs, without result. The whole upper leg shiny-red and hot; not the slightest touch could be endured; the child groans, and is in a continual fever, with profuse sweats, very much emaciated, and without any sleep and appetite.

I had the external application removed, and gave Silic. 30 in several doses. The child became more quiet and went to sleep. Some time afterwards a small opening formed spontaneously in the swelling, into which the thinnest probe could scarcely be introduced; there was a *thin* discharge from it, after which the opening closed up again. From this time on the boy improved rapidly (A. H. Z., 39, 2. H. Weber, of Brilon).

### 4. (C.) *Caries-Dyscrasia.*

A girl, æt. 8, could not straighten the left knee. Several fistulous ulcers upon it as well as on the lower leg. The tibia could be seen entirely denuded in several places, and smaller or larger pieces of it became detached. The whole tibia and knee was one single crusty ulcer almost, which bled on the slightest cause, and pained much, especially at night. Besides a few other remedies, the girl received *Calcar.* and *Silicea* for from three to four weeks. After the course of a year the crutches were laid aside, and gradually the whole leg healed. The crooked knee became straight and movable again, and at present the girl walks about as well as other people. No one would see that she ever had been sick (A. H. Z., 39, 19. Dr. Weber, of Brilon).

### 5. (CI.) *Eruption on the Face.*

Dr. Kämpfer (A. H. Z., 24, 10) reports a remarkable example of the great medicinal power of *Silicea.*

A woman, æt. 32, a blonde, who since childhood had suffered from a psoric-scrofulous ophthalmia, and against which she had formerly tried various cures, including homœopathic remedies, without result, was affected by an eruption of large, hard, brown crusts all over her lips, especially at the corners of the mouth, which very much disfigured the face. The eyes were almost entirely healthy. The remedies administered against it, among which was also *Silicea* 30, remained without any result.

I now prescribed *Silicea* 4, one drop to be taken every morning, and later every fourth morning before breakfast. She felt unwell every time after taking the medicine. After the first doses she was attacked by intense vertigo, violent headache with fulness and dulness in the head, heat and redness of the face, intense pain in the abdomen, nausea, heaviness in the limbs, feverish pulse, &c., so that she had to lie in bed for a few hours; affections she had never had before, and to which no cause could be assigned except the remedy, and which troubles always disappeared spontaneously. After the third dose these symptoms became lighter, and after the fourth she felt only fulness in the head and weakness. At the same time the eruption improved rapidly and without interruption, so that it healed up after five doses. The eyes and her general health continued to remain good. But soon afterwards a large and deep ulcer formed at the inside of the left lower leg, which continued for years.

It cannot be mistaken that the acute morbid phenomena, repeatedly appearing in this case after the remedy, were primary effects of the drug, and neither can it be doubted that the formation of the ulcer on the leg was owing to the action of the medicine (which has proved itself to me one of the most efficacious remedies against inveterate ulcers of this kind). Hence, in this case also, intense *remedial aggravations* took place, while high dilutions remained without any effect whatever. I have frequently made this observation, and could mention several similar cases.

NOTE.—With *Silicea* 3, I have repeatedly cured complaints that owed their origin to suppressed sweat of the feet.

*Nausea*, *fainting*, *weakness*, especially were complained of; hence, just the very symptoms called forth by *Silicea* 4, in Kämpfer's case. The sweat of the feet returned after the removal of the morbid phenomena mentioned.

### 6. (CII.) *Luxatio Spontanea.*

Dr. Weber, of Brilon (A. H. Z., 39, 2), reports: "A boy, æt. 8, from lying upon the damp ground in spring, was attacked by a fixed pain in the right *hip-joint; the leg shortened*, and patient began to limp. Soon afterwards the whole buttock swelled, the swelling, which is burning hot, extending down to the knees; patient has to lie down, and can lie only on the healthy side. Finally, the swelling threatened to break in several places, and to discharge the fluctuating contents.

"For this affection I treated patient for more than eight weeks. He received within this time Acon., Arnic., Arsen., Calcar., Chin., Hep. s., Lycopod., Phosph., Phosph. ac., Rhus, Sulphur, and *Silicea*. The latter remedy was given repeatedly. The swelling did not break but scattered entirely, and the boy was completely cured, and did not limp any longer. Every one who saw the swollen leg deemed resorption impossible; and yet it was possible, after all."

### 7. (CIII.) *Collection of Pus in the Cervical Glands and Lymphatic Swelling at the Elbow-Joint.*

#### TUMOR ALBUS.

A girl, æt. 15, a blonde, weakly formed, of phthisic habitus, and not menstruating yet, from her third year on frequently suffered from oft-recurring scrofulous glandular swellings. At her 9th year, without any cause known, a painful swelling of the left elbow-joint formed, which continued to grow for fully three years, and finally terminated in a painful hard swelling and anchylosis of the joint. After a pause of two years the pains returned, and the swelling began to enlarge again. Various cures tried against this trouble remained without any result. Lastly, on account of a fresh aggravation, warm applications and inunction of Iodine-salve were used; internally Kali hydrojod. in large doses. During this treatment, continued for two months, a considerable swelling of the right cervical glands formed again, swelling and pain increased, and the general health assumed a threatening aspect, which induced the parents to place patient under homœopathic treatment.

*Status præsens:* Patient is very much emaciated, has a pale face with circumscribed redness on the cheeks. Increased respiratory murmur; percussion normal. Transient stitches below both claviculæ. Dry, short cough, slight dyspnœa. Pulse very variable. At times febrile symptoms. The cervical glands of the right side had united into a swelling of the size of a hen's egg which was reddened and evenly fluctuating in its entire circumference. At the elbow-joint of the left arm a fluctuating swelling as large as a man's fist, which covered the olecranon partially, but the condylus humeri entirely. The forearm was bent at an angle of sixty degrees. On account of the great pain, the nights were passed sleepless; the stool was diarrhœic, especially at night.

The threatening development of acute pulmonary tuberculosis renders her condition very precarious.

Patient received now of Arsen. 15 ($\frac{1}{100}$) two doses daily, five pellets pro dosi.

Ten days later her general health improved somewhat. Arsen. was continued for other eight days, when the swelling at the joint broke in several places, and discharged a large quantity of thin, fluid pus and caseous masses. Since the chest symptoms had considerably improved. I gave *Silic.* 4 trit. ($\frac{1}{10}$) two grains of it daily, and ordered the arm to be bathed twice daily *in a decoction of hay. This popular remedy is probably efficacious* in scrofulous diseases, as I repeatedly had the opportunity of observing, *only on account of its contents of* TERRA SILICEA. This treatment was continued a whole year, during which time the complete cure of the arm, and the resorption of the swelling of the cervical glands were accomplished. The discharge of caseous masses which gave way, finally, to a serous secretion, continued for several months. The openings cicatrized and, with the exception of an insignificant swelling, no trace of a morbid state remained.

The mobility of the forearm has improved, since the angle of mobility now amounts only to $\frac{1}{10}$ degree. No trace is to be seen any longer of the (resorbed) swelling of the cervical glands (N. Z. f. h. Kl., 1, 6, Klinische Erfahrungen v. Dr. Hilberger, in Triest).

Davet (Journ. de la Soc. gall., III, 8, 1872) reports two cures of scrofula of the bone, which, although requiring some other remedies besides *Silicea*, would surely have been treated with far less success without it. Thus we better report them here:

### 8. (CIV.) *Caries of the Tarsal Joint and Bones of the Foot.*

Patient, æt. 20, upon whose foot the scrofulous affection had concentrated itself in consequence of luxation of the tarsal joint, for four years has not been able to put his foot down, and is cachectic in the highest degree. Around the diseased joint nine fistulous ulcerous openings. Great emaciation; grayish pale complexion; hectic fever; entire loss of appetite; now diarrhœa, now constipation; great irritability and sleeplessness.

*Silicea* 30, 15, and 200, in rare doses, continued for fifteen months (frequently with Nux vom. 6 as an intercurrent remedy against constipation; Arsen. against diarrhœa; Coffea against nervous irritability; and Ignatia when the latter increased to the development of phenomena resembling chorea) rapidly improved his condition, especially after a few bony splinters had been expelled, but did not effect cicatrization of the fistulous ulcers. This was accomplished two months later upon the continued administration of Argent. nitric. 3.

### 9. (CV.) *Gonarthrocace.*

In a boy, æt. 10, very much run down in flesh, a chronic osseous ulceration at the knee-joint of several years' standing was removed by Sil. 30 (together with Sulph., Asafœtid., Bellad , Merc. sol., Acid. nitri, as intercurrent remedies), and afterwards by *Silic.* in alternation with *Calc.* 30 within two years, while his general constitution was improved by sea-baths. The shortening of the leg, of course, remained.

### 10. (CVI.) *Luxatio spontanea femoris*

In consequence of preceding coxitis. Cured by Surgeon Schnappauf, of Dresden (Z. f. h. Kl. II, 9).

In an infant, seven months old, the femoral head had completely escaped out of the acetabulum and taken position posterio-superiorly; the leg was nearly one-twelfth of an inch shorter than the healthy one, yet not atrophic. Several physicians had declared the evil to be incurable on account of the acetabulum being filled up by exudations. When I reduced the femoral head and moved the extremity in various directions I distinctly heard a crackling and rubbing noise of the femoral head, entirely similar to that observed in fractures. As soon as the leg was released, and the child made a few motions with it, the femoral head again slipped out posteriorly with a crackling noise, without, however, causing the slightest painful sensation. The infant was a delicate but fleshy girl, and was nursed by her mother. In the first eight days after her birth, which had been natural and easy, a certain stiffness and immobility of the left leg had been observed; the babe always held it in a drawn-up position, and did not stretch it out even while being in the bath. Dr. K. declared the disease to be inflammation of the hip-joint. The entire region of the hip-joint was inflamed and swollen, a condition which had communicated itself also to the upper portion of the femur. An inunction had removed the inflammation, it is true, but now the femoral head was noticed to be outside of the acetabulum. Two experienced allopathic colleagues, in agreement with the first physician, declared that *nothing* could be done any more.

The attempts at reduction which Dr. K. daily made for some time, remained without permanent result. The advice of another physician, who ordered a pair of lace-boots, which sole side by side of sole were fastened to a tin plate, in hope that thus the healthy leg might draw down the diseased and keep it in the same position, proved also of no benefit to the affected extremity. This machine had almost occasioned another deformity, since the child, on account of the discomfort or pain originating therefrom, assumed a position inclining with the pelvis and vertebral column to the left side, for which reason the father of the child soon removed this contrivance.

Under such unfavorable circumstances the child was passed over to homœopathic treatment.

*Prescription: Silicea* 5 dil. from 2 to 3 drops to be taken in a teaspoonful of water every other evening. The child was not interfered with in its voluntary motions. After the course of five weeks no perceptible change in the condition had taken place, and the femoral head, after attempts at reduction, again slipped backward as on previous occasions. Notwithstanding, I continued *Silicea*, except that in place of the solution I gave the trituration in the same potency, because I presumed that in the trituration all the efficient constituents of the remedy were contained. This change was rewarded by the best result. After *Silicea* had been given in this manner for about three weeks, the crackling noise on moving the leg became slighter, the femoral head, after attempts at reposition, remained longer in the acetabulum, a fact which allowed the inference that the resorption of the hardened exudation had already begun. In order to support the soft tissue also, I ordered, at the intervals when no *Silic.* was taken, a teaspoonful of a mixture of one part of *Arnica fort.* to two parts of alcohol, to be rubbed into the region of the hip-joint and leg.

By the aid of these prescriptions, which I continued without alteration, I had the great pleasure of observing that the exudation was entirely resorbed at the latter part of January, and the femoral head, without any inclination to escape out of the joint upon motion and stepping on the foot, remained in the acetabulum, as well as that every noise had disappeared, of course, and could declare the child entirely cured at its first birthday, February 19th.

The author concludes his reports of this certainly highly instructive clinical observation with the following remark: "This cure has to be considered as the result of medical art all the more as the child meanwhile was carried about, and rest, which no doubt has effected a cure occasionally in single cases, was not observed in this one. An influence upon the main trouble could be attributed to the simultaneous use of Arnica all the less as the most evident signs of a beginning cure already appeared previously to it, and as such an influence upon cartilage and bone-tissue seems foreign to the action of Arnica, but is very characteristic of *Silicea.*

### 2. (CVII.) *Abscess.*

Dr. Billig, of Hohenstein (Z. f. h. Kl., 3, 8), reports a very remarkable result of the action of Silicea in a case of scrofulous suppuration. It was that of a boy, æt. 10, in whom, after recovery from typhus, an abscess developed. It opened at the right side of the thorax. From a fistulous opening at the place named, pus was discharged for three and a half years. Whenever the discharge stopped for a day or two, pain and dyspnœa set in. The fistulous character of the sinus, and the well-known power of *Silic.* in suppurations of various kinds, induced Dr. B. to give nine doses of *Silic.* 3, one grain pro dosi. These were consumed within the period of time from January 20 to February 6. Afterwards, six powders, with the direction to take one of the first three every third, of the remaining, one every fourth day. February 24th, the pus has become thinner and less. Six more powders, one from three to six days. They were the last given. Because suppuration soon ceased, the wound closed up without any complaints of the patient, similar to those previously experienced upon the arrest of the suppuration.

Against panaritia with which the scrofulous are so often afflicted, there is, aside from *Causticum* (Goullon), no better remedy than *Silicea.*

### 12. (CVIII.) *Thickening of the Last Phalanx of the Finger.*

A remarkable example of the amazing action of *Silicea* Kafka communicates (N. Z. f. h. Kl., 3, 4):

The last phalanx of the ring-finger of the right hand was

observed to be enlarged to double size; the skin around the edges of the nail is swollen, purple, and shiny; at both sides of the nail we see club-shaped, purple, and fleshy excrescences, as long as the nail, which nearly cover half of it with their broad, free surface, while, with their pedicle, they grow out of the side-walls of the matrix; the nails bleed very easily, and cause the most violent pain. Moreover, the nail over its whole length is undermined by pus, almost excavated underneath, and movable. Upon every motion or touch, indeed, even while at rest, throbbing and burning pains torture the patient during the day, which become unbearable at night, occasion sleeplessness, in consequence of which she looks very pale, and her appetite has become very poor.

The beneficial effect of *Silicea* 6 (morning and evening a powder, and externally white cerate), manifested itself as early as in the first night, since patient quietly slept several hours, and at waking up found the pains to be ameliorated in a high degree. Improvement progressed very rapidly; about six days later the excrescences looked shrunken and withered, were almost painless, and did not bleed any more. After other eight days the nail began to grow already, and after a treatment of three weeks the cure was accomplished, and a new, smooth, and pretty nail decorated the formerly diseased finger.

The woman had been under allopathic treatment for three months, and the nail was to be removed at the time she placed herself under homœopathic treatment.

### 13. (CIX.) *Panaritium.*

Dr. Eidherr, of Vienna, may be mentioned here as another authority. He says (N. Z. f. h. Kl., 5, 15):

No doubt every homœopathic physician has sufficiently experienced in his practice what value is to be ascribed to *Silicea* in diseases of the bones. I, at least, have learned its efficacy in *felons*, which were accompanied by the most violently stitching pains; in caries, and especially tumor albus, three cases of which I had the opportunity of observing within a very short time. I believe that *Silicea* in the disease-forms mentioned cannot be surpassed by any other remedy.

It is a peculiar fact that the most violent lancinating pains soon disappear after its administration. In caries I observed the carrion-like smell and ichorous discharge to give way very soon to a normal pus.

It seems that *Silicea*, from the very beginning, has to be given in all those cases of panaritium in which destruction of the bone (violent, nocturnal pains), can be proven. *Mercur.*, on the contrary, when the pains are not so violent, more throbbing than stinging, and the periosteum is not affected by the morbid process.*

14. (CX.)

Dr. Eidherr observed the same beneficial action of Silicea in *caries of the metatarsal bones*, and illustrates this observation by excellent examples (A. H. Z., 5, 14).

However, it may also happen that Silicea leaves us in the lurch. What then? Dr. Meyhoffer, of Nizza, reports an instructive case of this kind. The trouble, arising from scrofula, was caries of the epiphyses of the third, and, very probably, of the second cervical vertebræ. The surrounding soft tissues had become inflamed by the ulceration of the bone, and the pus broke through in an outward direction. At the left side of the spinal column a congestive abscess developing. Obsolete, tuberculous infiltration of the left pulmonary apex.

Mercur. bijodat. 0, 3, gr. 2, pro dosi.

November 4th. The discharge from the fistulous opening is very copious, but the pus better, creamy, and not so offensive any more.

November 10th. No further progress. Discharge of pus very considerable; the lower opening produced by a seton begins to cicatrize. Above the congestive abscess a slight arching of the skin may be noticed.

*Silicea* 0, 3, gr. 2, pro dosi, for eight days.

Nov. 20th. No essential change. Discharge of pus very profuse, the pain still considerable, the congestive abscess has arched out still more. Pulse 90, somewhat tense.

---

* See, however, under Mercur., cures of periostitis obtained by this remedy.

Since *Silicea* has had no effect, and the copious suppuration might exhaust the patient, Iodium was administered internally and externally.

℞. Iod. pur., gr. ii (0, 1)
Kali. hydroj., ℈j (1, 50)
Aqu. destil., ℥iv (120, 0)

Of this solution twenty drops were put into one-half litre of fresh water, and linen compresses dipped into it, wrung out, and laid on the congestive abscess and the swelling at the right side. In the same manner the lint was dipped in the same liquid. The compresses, when dry, were renewed. At the same time an injection was made into the fistulous ulcer every time after the evacuation of pus (tepid in place of cold water). The injected liquid remained in it from ten to twelve minutes. Internally Iod. 0, 3, gtt. 6 pro die. This was done till the end of November.

Nov. 30. The congestive abscess has disappeared entirely; the skin is livid on a small spot only, the pain has also ceased. The skin resumes its normal color. The edges of the fistulous opening are not callous any more, the spongy excrescences have disappeared and, at the bottom of the ulcer, we observe healthy granulation. *The purulent discharge is exceedingly small.* The right arm of the patient, which had become paretic, probably in consequence of the pressure of the inflamed soft tissue upon the dorsal nerves, is entirely relieved from this affection; appetite and sleep excellent.

Patient resumes work as a type-setter.

The same treatment is continued eight days longer, and since meanwhile the purulent discharge had stopped entirely, no more injections were made. The compresses are still continued; internally three drops of *Iod.* daily. At the end of December complete cicatrization of the ulcus fistulosum. The cure still continues a year afterwards.

### 15. (CXI.) *Caries cubiti sinistri cum anchylosi spuria.*

BY DR. MEYHOFFER, OF NIZZA.

Miss ——, for fifteen months suffering from an inflammation of the left elbow-joint, got steadily worse under the application of gray salve, local baths with sea-water, painting with Iodine, purgatives, and sulphur-waters (Challes in Savoy).

The inflammation is said to have originated without any perceptible cause. With the exception of measles and occasional slight *glandular swellings*, patient had been healthy thus far; menstruates regularly since her fourteenth year, and has a blooming appearance. The diseased arm is in a state of complete extension; neither active nor passive motions of flexion, supination, and pronation can be executed; every attempt at such calls forth the most violent pains in the cubital joint; the latter is considerably swollen and reddened at the inner as well as outer side; its temperature increased. The fossa supratrochlearis posterior has not only disappeared, but there is also a swelling in its place. At the condylus internus humeri a fistulous opening from six to eight millimetres in diameter, from which pale and spongy granulations sprout luxuriantly; from the opening a discharge of sanguino-serous pus in small quantities; the probe penetrates to the depth of one centimetre. Another fistulous opening can be seen in the centre of the olecranon from which very little serous pus is secreted; the probe on this spot, inwardly and upwardly penetrates the bone nearly to the depth of two centimetres.

Pain constant, but most violent in the evening, which probably may be accounted for by the tiring of the arm in consequence of its hanging position and the pressure of the exudation upon the nervus medianus.

The pathological process in this case has, hence, affected both epiphyses, and by the deposit of an exudation into the fossa cubiti anterior major, the introitus of the processus coronoideus has been rendered impossible.

In consideration of the inflammatory condition of the joint patient received (March 12th) Aconit. 0, 2 gtt. 6 pro die; absolutely horizontal position of the arm.

March 20th. The swelling of the joint considerably less, the redness almost entirely gone; no more spontaneous pain; the radius more free, slight passive motions of pronation and supination can be executed. The purulent discharge from both openings more copious and of a better quality.

*Silicea* 0, 3, one grain morning and evening; daily attempts at flexion. This treatment was continued a whole month, a pause of from three to four days being made after every six days' use of the remedy, as well as during menstruation.

April 25th. The forearm can be flexed without any pain so far as to form a right angle. The ulcer at the olecranon is cicatrizing. At the bottom of the ulcer healthy granulation.

Continuatur.

At the end of May even the fistulous opening at the condylus internus had healed by cicatrization, and Miss —— was able to flex her arm so far as to form an acute angle; in short, to execute any kind of motion with it (Z. f. h. Kl., 10, 20).

### 16. (CXII.) *Caries of the Femur and Tibia.*

Dr. Godée treated a scrofulous person, æt. 14, suffering from caries of the femur and the upper portion of the tibia. He received *Silicea* $\frac{6}{30}$ from six to eight days, according to the profuseness of the suppuration and detachment of the osseous fragments. He was told here that he could be cured only by an amputation of the leg. Indignant at this advice he returned to the former treatment, and was cured in ten months. Now twenty years of age, he enjoys the best of health (L'Hahnemannisme, 1868, No. 9; Silicea terra, Dr. Desterne).

Jousset calls *Silicea* le grand médicament de la scrofule. Should it, therefore, have no beneficial effect in scrofulous ophthalmia, which is the frequent expression of this dyscrasia? Dr. Schlosser, of Munich, may answer this question in place of us (A. H. Z., 56, 4).

### 17. (CXIII.) *Photophobia.—Perforating Ulcer on the Cornea.*

Linna H., æt. 7, of decidedly scrofulous constitution, a blue-eyed blonde, with delicate skin, since her vaccination has frequently been afflicted with cutaneous eruptions and ophthalmia. For six weeks she has suffered from photophobia, with pains in the eyes. On the right cornea an ulcer, with deeply imbedded bottom, and nearly perforating; considerable hyperæmia of the conjunctiva bulbi and eyelids; moist, vesicular eruption on the occiput.

Clematis 3, five pellets, twice a day, as well as Graphit. 12, remained without any effect.

One dose *Silicea* 200.

As early as in the evening patient complains less of pain. On the next morning she opened her eyes for the first time within seven weeks; simultaneously an exanthema, resembling measles, had broken out over her whole body during the night. The ophthalmic trouble remained cured; slight desquamation of the epidermis followed at the same time. The ulcer of the cornea so rapidly healed from the bottom and edges, and amid constant decrease of the conjunctivitis, that the effect of *Silic.* cannot be doubted.

### 18. (CXIV.) *Coxitis.*

The A. H. Z., 56, 9, among "Klinische Beobachtungen aus dem hom. Spitale in der Leopoldstadt zu Wien," contains a case of coxitis.

*Silicea*, it is said at the close, had a permanent effect. Though slowly, the pain nevertheless steadily decreased upon the continuation of the remedy until remarkable improvement had set in.

### 19. (CX.) *Caries of the Big Toe.*

G. B., of K., æt. 19, for more than a year suffered from caries of the right big toe. The physicians proposed the amputation of the toe as the only means to free him from his affliction. The toe was very thick, red, and swollen around the carious ulcer, so that he could not step on the foot. April 2d, *Silic.* 30. In June the toe was cured. Increased irritability in it again required *Silicea*, and August 14th patient wrote as follows: "I always think of you, and do not know what I ought to do to you out of gratitude for the delivery from my dangerous disease. I would never have believed that your powders, apparently a mere nothing, could produce such miracles."*

---

* Homöopath. Heilungen v. Dr. Kirsch, in Wiesbaden. A. H. Z., Bd. 79, No. 4.

### 20. (CXVI.) *Silicea against Nocturnal Convulsions of Scrofulous Children.*

(My own observation.)

An extraordinary, as well as sure curative action of *Silicea*, is the following:

E. B., a small, handsome, erethic-scrofulous boy, after having slept for an hour, suddenly wakes up amid distressing cries, jumps up, and cannot be appeased in less than half an hour. Trembling and spasmodic jerks of single groups of muscles remind one of the gesticulations of chorea minor. The agony forces the sweat out of the pores. At the same time he has the sensation as if something crawled over his face, and he repeatedly attempts to grasp it. Presence of ascarides proven. They have kept quiet, however, lately. These attacks, daily recurring for three weeks, forthwith ceased after the first dose of a solution of *Silicea* 30 (2 drops in 12 teaspoonfuls of water, morning and evening a teaspoonful).

---

Finally, a few clinical hints from Rückert's "Attempt at utilizing the curative material obtained *ab usu in morbis:*"

The percentage of Terra silicea contained in so many mineral springs, and thus far overlooked, is to be rated higher, since several of them owe their character to this constituent.

v. Grauvogl mentions *Silicea* as a nutrition remedy among the series of substances against the *hydrogenoid* constitution. It certainly has very special bearings upon the organs of the vegetative system.

Aggravation of the whole morbid condition when the moon is waxing.

Constitution feeble; skin thin, delicate; face pale.

Moreover, the fact that nutrition is poor, not, however, in consequence of poor food, but deficient assimilation (such persons are usually constipated), argues in favor of the importance of *Silicea* as an antiscrofulosum. Quiet sleep is a contraindication to *Silicea*.

Again *Silicea* deserves the rank of a specific against hæmatoma cerebrale.

Its indications, corroborated as they have been in diseases of the eye, are valuable: Swelling of the right saccus lacrymalis; the discharged tears are hot.

In the gravest affections of the most various kind, especially in ophthalmia, when perforation of the cornea threatens, in ulcerations of the cornea with swelling of the lids, if it has become chronic and painful.

Formation of abscesses of the size of a lentil in the upper part of the iris appearing as yellowish-red swellings, covering the entire pupil. The pus, a portion of which has escaped into the anterior eye-chamber, was entirely removed.*

Sensation as from smoke or mist before the eyes. Eyes inflamed, red, and watering. An unmistakable, intense, and grayish turbidity of the crystalline lens of the right eye was removed so far as to leave but a very minute small speck.

Complete cure of a gray cataract of more than one year's standing by *Silicea*, one dose every month.

In dysekoia and amblyopia of sensitive persons.

A woman got rid of the sweat of the feet, but was afflicted in consequence by a decrease of the power of vision so that she could see but capitals. The sweat of the feet having returned upon taking *Silicea*, she sees better now than before.†

Scrofulous otorrhœa of several years' standing, offensive, with soreness of the inner nose and a crusty eruption on the upper lip.

For scrofulous and rhachitic persons whose teeth are mostly carious and necrotic, and when the toothache aggravates, especially at night and on inhaling cold air.

The throbbing toothache cured by *Silicea* is connected with swelling of the periosteum or the lower jaw itself; the pain is seated more in the latter than in the tooth, and sleep is disturbed on account of general heat.

Spitting of a viscid and mucous saliva is frequently connected therewith; profuse secretion of saliva indicating *Silicea* all the more. Here we observe a relation to Mercur., with which remedy, moreover, *Silicea* has in common the name of

---

* Senega is also recommended for the resorption of hypopia.

† I recollect a similar cure with Silicea, in which, according to report, the hearing of the ear previously diseased became better than that of the healthy ear.

a toothache remedy. This may also be said of Arsen. All three frequently relieve the sleeplessness of persons afflicted with toothache, which tortures them to desperation almost.

If resorption cannot be expected any more in tonsillitis, the tongue is thickly coated, and the face distorted spasmodically while swallowing, *Silicea* rapidly matures and cures the abscess.

It is also suitable if the throat, without being inflamed, pains on swallowing.

Further, in scrofulous swelling and induration of the cervical glands, in parotitis, gradually developing, slowly increasing, very chronic, frequently attaining to an enormous size, nearly without pain, redness and heat of the skin. (See also Cure III, Lycopod.)

Again, in malignant scrofulous ulcers and fistulous sinuses of the lymphatic cervical glands, and caries of the clavicula.

Finally, panaritia (p. cutaneum, p. tendinosum, and p. periosticum), so frequent among the scrofulous, as well as the carbuncle at the neck, offer excellent opportunities to convince us of the specific curative action of *Silicea*.

NOTE 1.—Dr. A. R., of S., reports: "I have not known that *Silicea* is also a popular remedy. In this section of the country the inhabitants use the fine dust of a pebble, the so-called '*Teufelsfinger*' (*devil's-finger*), against ulcers and suppurating wounds. It is a very hard, blackish, and smooth stone, of elongated form, somewhat resembling a finger. It is scraped, the powder being strewed upon the suppurating spot. I have been told that frequent cures of old, malignant sores have been accomplished by it" (A. H. Z., März, 1869).

NOTE 2.—*Kaoline*, potentized porcelain-earth, recently often mentioned in the A. H. Z., is related to Silic.* October 4th, 1869, Dr. Landesmann, of Geneva, published a few interesting cures of croup by Kaoline 6. It helped in the very worst cases in which Acon., Hep. sulph., Spong., Brom., Phosph., and Iodium had failed.

Shortly afterwards the homœopathic veteran Aegidi claimed

* Kaoline is a Silicate of Alumina $= Al^3 S^3 + 6H$.

the priority of this remedy, stating that, at a much earlier date, he had obtained excellent results with it (the 6th and 30th), in croup.

Landesmann finds Kaoline indicated if the seat of the croupous inflammation is in the lower portion of the larynx, and the upper portion of the trachea, a condition which may be diagnosticated from the much more laborious and sawing inspiration, experiencing an impediment just at this spot, situated lower down.

Since, especially, the most grave cases of croup coincide with scrofulosis, we take notice here of these observations of Landesmann and Aegidi.*

## SPONGIA TOSTA.

### GENERALITIES.

Is Spongia a remedy against scrofulosis? Certainly not in the same sense as Sulph., Calc. carb., Phosph., and others are. It undoubtedly enjoys its most extensive fame in croup, yet the cases ought to be strictly individualized, since examples are known in which *Spongia* surely did not accomplish anything. The beneficial influence exerted by sponges, dipped into hot water and applied to the throat of croup patients, most surely is not foreign to the antiscrofulous action of *Spongia*. Its curative action upon strumatous swellings, which, as is well known, in former times were identified with scrofulosis, hence, the former name struma for scrofula is just as certain. For this very reason the remedy, also designated as "Kropf-Schwamm," rightfully claims its place among the series of antiscrofulosa. However, we shall be less surprised at the excellent effects of *Spongia* in scrofulous processes, if we consider that it contains Iod., Sulph., Phosph., Kali hydrojod., Kali bromic., and Carbo veget. It is not improbable, that the greater or less reliability of the remedy in croup depends upon the various quantitative proportion of these substances. By this, its *modus operandi* upon the glandular

* Here we will remind our esteemed colleague, Aegidi, of his promise to give us other clinical hints for the administration of Kaoline.

system may also be explained. Aside from its action upon the thyroid gland, its influence upon the testes (in orchitis), is unmistakable.

### CLINIQUE.

#### 1. (CXVII.) *Croup.*

Bolle, of Paderborn (A. H. Z., 48, 8), reports two interesting cures of croup, from which he infers that *Spongia*, by itself, cures not only fresh, but also neglected cases. "I could," he continues, "mention still many more fresh and neglected cases which were cured by me with *Spong.* 3. It would be of no interest, however, to do so, since one case of angina membran. too much resembles the other, in order to find it worth while to report them separately."*

#### 2. (CXVIII.)

Dr. Billig cured his own blooming boy, five years old, who was attacked by croup, with *Tinct. Spongiæ* alone (gtt. vj to a cupful of water, two teaspoonfuls from ¼ to 1 hour) (A. H. Z., 44, 22).

## SULPHUR.

### GENERALITIES.

"After Serapion, of Alexandria, 270 A.C., had discovered Sulphur as the specific against chronic cutaneous eruptions, it was used and praised in all its preparations for centuries, to the most recent times."

The great range of the curative action of *Sulphur* can be explained only by the aid of Hahnemann's psora-hypothesis, which, taken *cum grano salis*, allows a deep insight into the inner nature of many *chronic* diseases. For seven-eighths of the latter, according to Hahnemann's researches, owe their origin, and especially their obstinacy to this cause. By psora

* Bolle gives 1 gr. of Spong. 3, and then waits for another spell of cough before administering a second dose.

we do not understand, however, the eruption produced by the acarus, but the sum of certain biological obstacles which resist, deface, and complicate the natural course of diseases. These hindrances do not refer to the phenomena comprised by the term "*syphilitic*," but, on the contrary, occupy a position opposite thereto.

The constitutional conditions of our ancestors play, probably, the principal part in the appearance of psora. For, in the same manner as mental deficiencies and anomalies are transferred to us from our parents, grandparents, and ancestors far more remote, so their physical deficiencies, though modified, are also transferred to us; hence, mental and physical tendencies.*

It is of practical importance to abandon the division of chronic diseases into two large classes (psora and syphilis, to which, as the third, we must properly add sycosis) and, according to the name of the specific remedy eradicating the disease, to speak of Sulphur-psora, Arsenic-psora, Phosphor-Silicea-psora, &c.

So many "*antipsorica*," so many "*psora species*."

Without these remedies no chronic psora-disease is ever cured. On the contrary, however, innumerable other non-psoric (non-syphilitic and non-sycotic) diseases heal spontaneously by proper diet and manner of living (a fact that was known to Hahnemann as well as to the more recent physiological school).

The great merit of the introduction of psora, in our opinion, consists in this, that, by means of it, the connection of *certain* (not of all) processes on the skin (the mucous membranes included) with the entire organism has been fixed for all time to come, and the doctrine of the local nature of cutaneous eruptions has been completely overthrown.

Virchow's remark, "The parasitic acari may pass through their whole development on a human being, they may copulate, lay eggs, and the offspring may be developed without any perceptible trace whatever of scabies in some persons" (Handbuch der Pathologie und Therapie, 1, 471), presents a

---

* Among the primary groups of psora-symptoms, the so-called "Grindkopf" has received the name of "Erbgrind," not accidentally, perhaps.

brilliant proof of the acarus becoming only the occasional cause of awakening the slumbering disease (the slumbering psora-poison) which, otherwise, might probably not have manifested itself before months or years, or even not at all.

And now we will pass on to "*Sulphur-psora*," and thus to the relations of *Sulphur* to scrofulosis.

Since *Sulphur* in its principal physiological action affects the venous system, it becomes the most excellent scrofula-remedy. It is specific in all *scabious* forms of cutaneous eruptions, of which scrofulosis can exhibit so many without any dependence of the eruption upon the presence of parasites.* The therapeutic bearing of Sulphur to the glandular system becomes plain from the fixed fact that it affects the *whole lymphatic system* as well as *all secreting surfaces* and, hence, also the glands, and has been employed with the best results in diseases that have taken root there (Reil).

*Sulphur* removes troubles of the respiratory organs (hoarseness, blennorrhœa pulmonum, difficult respiration, asthmatic affections, symptoms of incipient *phthisis pulmonum*—condensation of the pulmonary tissue in the apices; irritation in the larynx, dry cough), the more easily, the more plainly the scrofulous habitus is associated with the symptoms mentioned.

The same holds good of aphthæ, panaritia, inflammation of the eyelids, photophobia, &c., finally of the swellings of the lips, nose, submaxillary glands and tonsils so suitable for *Sulphur*.

What an immense difference between the vague recommendation of laxants consisting of calomel and jalap, or of teas said to purify the blood, or cures with Cod-liver oil, &c., and the recommendation of *Sulphur*, incomparably more clear and sure, where it is indicated homœopathically. Within the firmly fixed sphere of its positive, curative power belong, moreover: Crusta lactea; tinea capitis humida, ophth. scroful. (ulcera corneæ), ophth. neonat. (here especially Hepar sulph. c.), otorrhœa scrof., rhachitic affections, and such complaints especially as owe their origin to an irrational removal of exanthematous affections, *i. e.*, of peripheric curative at-

* Scabies of a *pointed form*, according to Heichelheim, was not cured by Sulphur.

tempts of the vital forces. (See CXXIII.) Thus *Sulphur* (as does Graphit.) restores the hæmorrhoidal flow. Insufferable itching is characteristic of *Sulphur* (especially at night), if we wish to cure an existing exanthema; but eruptions "*of all kind*" are not suitable for it.

### CLINIQUE.

#### 1. (CXIX.) *General Scrofulosis.*

A boy, 1½ year old, descending from scrofulous parents and himself scrofulous in a high degree, suffering from swellings of the cervical glands, ulcers and inflammation of the eyelids, has been treated allopathically for a long time by Baryt. mur., Kal. hydroj., Digitalis, Conium mac., and salves of red precipitate and zinc, and since all this proved of no avail, by Calomel in pretty large doses, and afterwards Iodine. Finally, my advice was requested, and I found a real picture of misery; the child seemed to be doomed to die without any possible hope of saving it. The boy was not able to walk yet. The whole neck was covered partly with open, glandular swellings discharging a thin, yellow liquid; partly with such as threatened to break; the crusty ears discharged, and diffused a very offensive smell. The eyelids were swollen and inflamed, the cornea opaque, and covered with cicatrices and fresh ulcers; the scalp was overspread by stinking crusts; profuse flow of saliva constantly tormented the patient, and intense, hectic fever, accompanied by a dry cough, had exhausted all vital power and produced great emaciation.

In view of these conditions, I could not prognosticate favorably, and advised the father better not to begin another cure, but to leave everything to nature. But he would not consent to this, and thus I prescribed *Tinct. Sulphuris* 1, and ordered one drop of it to be given morning and evening.

A good while afterwards I was not a little surprised upon hearing that gradually everything had improved, the ulcers had healed by and by, and the boy was now entirely well, and nobody able to imagine his former condition from his present appearance. Entirely satisfied with the result, they had not deemed it necessary to give any more medicine (A. H. Z., 60, 22).

2. (CXX.)

*Spirit. Sulphuris*, within fourteen days, cured a gray cataract which had developed after driving away a crusty eruption on the head (A. H. Z., 55, 3).

Dr. Eidherr, in cases in which the internal administration of *Sulphur* led to no result, uses with the best success the tincture of *Sulphur** of which a few drops were put into water, as a wash (A. H. Z., 60, 12).

3. (CXXI.) *Ophthalmia Scrofulosa.*

Caroline H., of W., æt. 5, of scrofulous diathesis, at the end of 1840 was attacked by scrofulous ophthalmia, against which the parents had sought the advice of a few allopathic physicians. The child had taken a good deal of Mercury, but was not cured.

*Status præsens:* Only the right eye is affected. Photophobia in a slight degree; several red vessels traverse the eye, especially from below toward the cornea on which a nubecula can be observed. The child complains sometimes of pain in the eye, and is sad and depressed, as the scrofulous mostly are.

*Sulphur* (gtt. i, dil. 3, pulv. iii, every fourth day), *Bellad.* (gtt. i, dil. 3, pulv. viii, one a day), again *Sulphur* (gtt. i, dil. 3, pulv. iii, every fourth day), and finally *Calc. carb.* (gtt. i, dil. 4, pulv. xii, one every other day), completely cured the

---

* *Spiritus Sulphuris.* Mr. Peters, the apothecary, writes Rummel, a short time ago, showed me a *Spirit. Sulph.*, which he had prepared at first by a careful trituration of *Sulphur* alone and then with alcohol, and which manifested itself already by its sensible properties as an exceedingly powerful preparation. For, a few drops of it put into water developed the smell of *Sulphur* so intensely that all doubt as to its solubility in alcohol is removed. Hence, we see how much a careful trituration adds to the development of medicinal forces, how much, moreover, is depending upon the proper preparation, and how important it is to procure medicines only from reliable pharmacies, or to prepare them ourselves. At the same time he expresses the wish to prepare Mercur., Carb. veg., Graph., Silic., &c., in the same manner (A. H. Z., 11, 11).

child within a short time* (Bd. xxi, No. 19, Beobachtungen und Erfahrungen aus der Praxis v. Dr. Frank).

4. (CXXII.) *Scrofulous Eruption.*

A boy, three years of age, pot-bellied, with pustules and herpetic crusts in the face, around the ear, and on the hairy scalp; a swelling as large as a pigeon's-egg, dark-red, elastic, and painful, on which a punctum suppurativum could be seen, and disturbed general health, was cured within ten days by *Sulphur*, a dose every other day.

(I wonder whether the favored laxantia and the Pulv. alterans Plummeri, which is said to have helped frequently, would have effected a cure of the eruption as rapidly and pleasantly as *Sulphur* indicated here? Counting eczema among the most benignant forms of cutaneous eruptions, we are notwithstanding told by Schönlein that in the majority of cases the disease lasts from six to seven weeks. Rep.) (Hygea 15, 3 Heft.)

5. (CXXIII.) *Otorrhœa.*

In another case *Sulphur* 3, a dose every other day, within six days cured a purulent, offensive otorrhœa, with discharging crusts behind the ears (Ibidem).

6. (CXXIV.)

*Three panaritia and a digital ulcer*, treated partly by poultices, partly with salves and knife, were rapidly cured by *Silicea* and *Sulphur*, in which cures the speedy removal of the pains proved itself an especial blessing (Ibidem).

7. (CXXV.)

Rückert cured with *Sulph.* 30 and 2, two cases of ophthalmia neonatorum (N. f. h. Kl., 5, 22).

---

* In this case we deem the simultaneous application of Calc. carb. unessential.

## 8. (CXXVI.)

A child, æt. 3, which in the first year of its life had suffered from crusta lactea, and afterwards from a febrile condition, had a stupid look, permanent diarrhœa, and was emaciated to an enormous degree. Œdema of the extremities, ascites, ferocious appetite, thirst, and lentescent fever.

*Arsen.* 30, three doses, within two days decreased the fever, thirst, and diarrhœa. During the following eight days the child received no medicine. No change.

Now *Sulphur* one dose in twenty-four hours.

Fourteen days afterwards the little patient could hardly be recognized; he was cured. Watering of the eyes and constipation, which had remained, gave way within a month to *Sulph.* and *Calc.*, so that somewhat later the child enjoyed complete health (Espanet.-Journal de la Societé Gallic. de Méd. hom., 15 Nov., 1857).

## 9. (CXXVII.) *Scrofulous Eruption.*

Dr. Cohnfeld (Berlin) found *Sulphur* efficacious in all forms of eruptions with the exception of the syphilitic and the ringworm. He, therefore, calls *Sulphur* (and *Arsen.*) the apostles who converted him, truly and radically, since by the irresistible force of facts they eradicated the skepsis with which, as a disciple of chemico-physical science, he arraigned himself against homœopathy, and especially against the doctrine of potencies.

The indication for *Sulphur* in eruptive diseases, more limited, as it is, becomes plain from a case of the same author which we report here.

The son of a laborer, æt. 5, is covered over the whole face with a coppery-red, shiny, and crusty tinea, which is overflooded here and there by a greenish ichor. He has scratched in several places bleeding sores in the disgusting mask, which render his appearance still more hideous. The body of the child, not too much emaciated, was covered with crusts and crusty herpetic spots, varying from the size of a dime to that of the palm of the hand. The disease had appeared three months after birth, had developed itself within a year or so to its present height, and *existed to this extent nine months.* Besides large quantities of Cod-liver oil, all allopathic remedies had been used, without, however, effecting an amelioration of the evil, even.

Four powders of *Sulph.* 30, one every third day.

Fourteen days later, says Dr. C., the woman returned with another boy who likewise suffered from tinea faciei, though of a very slight nature. It consisted in dry, red, herpetic spots on cheeks and forehead, and a small discharging spot on the chin. Above all I inquired how the other patient was. "Well," said the woman, "he is better, as you see." As I see! The woman had to assure me repeatedly that the boy before me looking like a human being was the frightful sight I had seen fourteen days ago. The remedy is repeated, and in another fortnight the face was completely clean and healthy.

The crusty herpes upon the body considerably diminished. After four more doses of *Sulph.* the whole eruption had disappeared, with the exception of a few crusts. The *propter hoc*, Cohnfeld concludes this interesting report, in which every word is conviction, cannot be subjected to any doubt in this case* (A. H. Z., 60, 25).

We will yet mention that C., in his recommendation of Sulphur and Arsen., has in view the higher potencies. Dr. Freitag (Leipzig) also says (where he speaks of the nature and treatment of scabies, A. H. Z., 60, 9): "*Sulphur, in the higher potencies, always seemed to me to act more favorably than in the lower.*"

From this very able article we will quote yet the following passage, deserving our consideration:

"Every homœopathic physician, industrious in his researches, and impartial in his observations, will be able to adduce examples which show that upon the internal use of

* Dr. I. O. Müller is of the opinion "that the external application of Sulphur, in fresh, genuine itch, can be made without any harm, and that only those forms have to be excluded, probably, the *duration of which for years* proves a relation (which cannot be defined more precisely though) between the affection and the entire organism, in which case, then, the internal treatment offers results all the more satisfactory." Cohnfeld's case belongs here.

the antipsorica, so called, especially of *Sulphur*, eruptions of the most various kind develop, eruptions by the appearance of which a gradual cure of the diseased inner organ is initiated. I have seen such very extraordinary results obtained by the homœopathic method of healing in inveterate and neglected cases of eczema, lichen, prurigo, &c., dependent upon scabies driven away previously. Cases which, for years, resisted all the artificially compounded washes and salves of allopathic physicians, gave way within months to the (so-called) antipsorica employed without any external medicines whatever having been administered as aids. And here *Sulphur*, again, is an inestimable remedy.

NOTE 1.—Scrofulous troubles (especially among children) in which the eye seems to be affected little proportionally (the eyes are somewhat red, hardly agglutinate, and show but a slight degree of photophobia), but a formation of small pustules takes place at the temporal region, and around the eye, are cured, even after a duration of years, in a short time, by *Sulph.* 3, a dose every evening (A. H. Z., 77, 10).

NOTE 2.—*Sulphur* deserves consideration in *fluent* coryza with spasmodic sneezing, intense catarrh of the choanæ, in which the nasal discharge is frequently intermixed with blood; in hoarseness, with a rough bass voice, dryness in the throat, and burning on swallowing (Kafka).

*Sulphur* affords help yet in neglected cases of chronic coryza (Bär).

---

## TEUCRIUM MARUM VERUM.

### GENERALITIES.

Against nasal polypi, and the catarrhal discharge dependent thereupon (Dr. Black, Brit. Journ. of Hom., Apr., 1857). Especially against mucous polypi (Kopp). We must not overlook this remedy on account of its action upon the nasal mucosa, though we may not be justified, on the other hand, to count it among the most approved antiscrofulous remedies.

Besides, *Teucrium* is used against ascarides, the presence of which so frequently coincides with the scrofulous habitus.

Of the remedial effects pertaining here we name: Headache; dulness of the head; pressing in the forehead above the eyes; eyes red and inflamed, accompanied by coryza; violent sneezing; great obstruction in the nose; dry cough, with tickling in the trachea.

### CLINIQUE.

#### 1. (CXXVIII.) *Polypi.*

Dr. Tuwar, of Prague, reports a case, in which nasal polypi were removed by painting with *Tinct. Teucrii mar. ver.* In similar cases *Teucrium* was also used in the form of snuff (as errhinum).

#### 2. (CXXIX.) *Polypi.*

Dr. Rhees (Amer. Hom. Review) reports:

A woman, æt. 25, had a polypus in the right cavity of the nose, which had been removed by an operation twice within the last three years, but in consequence of coryza had re-formed again for the third time. Patient felt tickling and painful pricking at the root of the nose, and in the left frontal protuberance. The eye watered, and much mucus is discharged from the left nasal cavity. Blowing the nose occasions pain, and occasionally hemorrhage. She can inhale only through the right nasal cavity. *Teucrium* 6, twice a day, for fourteen days remained without result. Now the 1st dilution was given for one week, in the second week the 3d dilution, and in the third week again the 1st dilution. Hereupon decrease of the polypus in size, and decrease of the mucous discharge. Air can pass through the left nasal cavity. During the next week the same prescription. After that the polypus had disappeared, and patient experienced only an unpleasant feeling in the left nasal cavity, which soon disappeared, however. Four years later, in consequence of coryza, patient was affected by obstruction of the left nasal cavity and occasional pricking at the root of the nose, yet an examination did not disclose anything. This trouble disappeared after the first dose of *Teucrium* 6.

### 3. (CXXX.) *Polypi.*

In the Hygea, Veith reports the cure of a nasal polypus by *Teucrium.* And, in the same manner, Dr. Hermel cured one by *Teucr.* 3 (2 drops in 200, 0 of water, morning and evening a spoonful). L'Art. Méd., Nov., 1858. We repeat that other remedies have relations much more specific to the scrofula-process itself, and hence come into consideration in cases of polypus upon purely scrofulous bottom. Among these *Calc. carb.* especially belongs.

As regards external applications in the treatment of polypi, we deem it in place to say that polypi of the meatus audit. ext. were also cured in the same manner; but in these cases it was not done by Tinct. Teucr., but by *Tr. Opii*, in its remedial relation very different, no doubt, from the former* (Rainer).

### 4 and 5. (CXXXI and CXXXII.)

Dr. Gabaldo also cured a nasal polypus with *Teucrium* 12, and afterwards T. 24, and Dr. Roth a pear-shaped, soft, and flat polypus, five inches in length, protruding from the vaginal opening in a girl 25 years of age (L'Art. Méd., Nov., 1858, in A. H. Z., 58, 4).

---

## VIOLA TRICOLOR, IACEA.

### GENERALITIES.

Stark regards it a specific against crusta lact. Although, aside from its action upon the urinary organs, intestinal tract and skin, the secretion of which it increases, it affects the

* As early as in 1809, Primus cured an aural polypus by applying to it lint saturated with Tr. Opii several times a day. As early as after a few days the polypus very perceptibly decreased in size, and eight days later fell off spontaneously as a dried up, skinny concrement. In the cases observed by Rau the polypus withered much more slowly, and did not become detached before several weeks.

lymphatic system also; the indication for it, nevertheless, appears to have been based upon too general grounds. How often, on receiving scrofulous patients, must we hear the answer to the question, "Have you given the child something already?" "Yes, we did let it drink *pancey tea.*" It is a fact, however, that the provings of Hahnemann, Franz, Wislicenus a. o., mention as special remedial effect, "Eruption with nightly itching, and dense, thick crusts in the face, from which a yellow pus discharges."

### CLINIQUE.

#### 1. (CXXXIII.) *Crusta lactea.*

A girl, six years old, for weeks suffered from scrofulous ophthalmia of both eyes. The face was covered formerly with a dry, and now, in consequence of poultices, discharging crusta lactea. *Viol. tr.* caused the eruption to become dry again, and cured it within three weeks. The eyes improved with the disappearance of the eruption (Z. f. h. Kl., 2, 21).

# RÉSUMÉ OF CURES REPORTED.

## *A.*—SKIN.

| | | |
|---|---|---|
| XXXIX. | Impetigo figurata, . . . | Calc. carb. |
| LI. | Pemphigus, . . . . . | Dulcamara. |
| LVII. | Eczema capitis, . . . . | Hep. sulph. calc. |
| LXX. | Eczema rubrum, . . . . | Ferrum jodat. |
| LXXV. | Eczema capitis et faciei, . . | Kali chrom. |
| LXXVIII. | Verrucæ, . . . . . . | Lycopodium. |
| LXXXVI. | Eczema impetiginodes, . . | Mercur. |
| CI. | Eruption on the face, . . . | Silicea. |
| CXII. | Impetigo capitis, . . . . | Sulphur. |
| CXXVII. | Impetigo larvata, . . . | Sulphur. |
| CXXXIII. | Crusta lactea, . . . . . | Viola tricolor. |
| XLIX. | Abscess on the lower leg, . . | Silicea. |
| CVII. | Abscess, . . . . . . | Silicea. |

## *B.*—EYES.

| | | |
|---|---|---|
| I. | Ophthalmia scrofulosa, . . | Acid. nitri. |
| II. | Blepharitis phlegmonosa, . . | Acid. nitri. |
| III. | Ophthalmia scrofulosa, . . | Apis. |
| IV. | Ophthalm. scroful., . . . | Apis. |
| VIII. | Ophthalm. scroful., . . . | Arsen. |
| IX. | Ophthalm. scroful., . . . | Arsen. |
| X. | Ophthalm. scroful., . . . | Arsen. |
| XV. | Keratitis chronica, . . . | Aurum. |
| XVI. | Keratit. chronic., . . . | Aurum. |
| XVII. | Ophthalm. rheumatico-scrof., . | Aurum. |
| XX. | Ophthalm. scroful., . . . | Baryt. mur. |
| XXXVIII. | Ophthalm. scroful., . . . | Calc. carb. |
| XLV. | Blepharoblennorrhœa, . . . | Calc. carb. |

LII. Spots on the cornea, . . . Euphrasia.
LIII. Opacities of the cornea, . . Euphrasia.
LIV. Ophthalm. scroful., . . . Hepar.
LVI. Ophthalm. neonatorum, . . Hepar.
LVIII. Ophthalm. scroful., . . . Hepar.
LXXXI. Ophthalm. scroful., . . . Mercur.
XCVI. Ophthalm. scroful., . . . Rhus.
CXVI. Ulcus corneæ perforans, . . Silicea.
CXX. Cataract after suppressed tinea, . Spir. sulph.
CXXI. Ophthalm. scroful., . . . Sulphur.
CXXV. Ophthalm. neonat., . . . Sulphur.

## *C.*—EARS.

XXXIV. Otorrhœa, . . . . . . Calc. carb.
LXXXII. Otorrhœa, . . . . . . Merc. solub.
CXXIII. Otorrhœa, . . . . . . Sulphur.

## *D.*—NOSE.

XIII. Ozæna,. . . . . . . Aurum.
XIV. Ozæna,. . . . . . . Aurum.
XXXVI. Polypus, . . . . . . Calc. carb.
XXXVII. Polypus, . . . . . . Calc. carb.
XLVI. Fibrous polypus, . . . . . Calc. carb.
LXXII. Coryza chronica, . . . . . Kali bichrom.
LXXIV. Coryza chron., . . . . . Kali bichrom.
LXXVI. Coryza chron., . . . . . Kali bichrom.
LXXXVII. Coryza chron., . . . . . Natrum carb.
LXXXVIII. Coryza chron., . . . . . Natrum carb.
CXXVIII. Polypus, . . . . . . Teucrium.
CXXIX. Polypus, . . . . . . Teucrium.
CXXX. Polypus, . . . . . . Teucrium.
CXXXI. Polypus, . . . . . . Teucrium.*

## *E.*—MOUTH.

LXXIII. Aphthæ, . . . . . . Mercurius.

---

* CXXXII. Polypus vaginæ.

## *F.*—GLANDS.

| | | |
|---|---|---|
| XXVII. | Mesenterial glands, . . . | Bromium. |
| XXVIII. | Cervical " . . . | " |
| XXIX. | " " . . . | " |
| XXX. | Amygdalitis chronica, . . . | " |
| XXXI. | Submaxillary glands, . . . | " |
| XXXII. | " " . . . | " |
| L. | Hypertrophical gland, . . . | Conium. |
| LIX. | Axillary gland, . . . . | Hep. sulph. calc. |
| LXXVIII. | Hypertrophia of the tonsil, . . | Kali chrom. |
| LXXX. | Cervical glands, . . . . | Lycopodium. |
| LXXXIV. | Angina tonsillaris, . . . | Mercurius. |

### CURES OF STRUMATA.

| | | |
|---|---|---|
| V. | Struma, . . . . . . | Apis. |
| VI. | " . . . . . . . . | " |
| VII. | " . . . . . . . . | " |
| XLI. | " . . . . . . . . | Calc. carb. |
| XLII. | " . . . . . . . . | " " |
| XLIII. | " . . . . . . . . | " " |
| IX. | " . . . . . . . . | Iodium. |
| LXVIII. | " . . . . . . . . | Kali hydrojod. |

## *G.*—BONES AND JOINTS.

| | | |
|---|---|---|
| XXV. | Gonarthrocace, . . . . | Calc. carb. |
| XLVII. | Spondylarthrocace, . . . | " " |
| LXVII. | Coxarthrocace, . . . . | Ol. jec. as. |
| LXXXV. | Periostitis, . . . . . | Mercurius. |
| XCV. | Luxatio spontanea, . . . | Rhus. |
| XCVII. | Caries of the right metatarsal bones, . . . . . . | Silicea. |
| XCVIII. | Spondylarthrocace, . . . | " |
| C. | Dyscrasia cariosa, . . . | " |
| CII. | Luxatio spontanea, . . . | " |
| CIII. | Tumor albus, . . . . | " |
| CIV. | Caries of the tarsal joint, . . | " |
| CV. | Gonarthrocace, . . . . | " |

| | | |
|---|---|---|
| CVI. | Luxatio spontanea, . . . | Silicea. |
| CVIII. | Thickening of phalanx, . . | " |
| CIX. | Panaritium, . . . . . | " |
| CX. | Caries of the metatarsal bones, . | " |
| CXI. | Caries of the elbow-joint, . . | " |
| CXII. | " femoris, . . . . . | " |
| CXIII. | Coxitis, . . . . . . | " |
| CXV. | Caries of the big toe, . . . | " |

## *H.*—LARYNX.

### CURES OF CROUP.

| | | |
|---|---|---|
| XXI. | Croup, . . . . . . . | Bromium. |
| XXII. | " . . . . . . . | " |
| XXIII. | " . . . . . . . | " |
| XXV. | " . . . . . . . | " |
| XXVI. | " . . . . . . . | " |
| LV. | " . . . . . . . | Hep. sulph. calc. |
| LXI. | Asthma laryngeum, . . . | Iodium. |
| LXII. | Croup, . . . . . . . | " |
| LXIII. | " . . . . . . . | " |
| LXIV. | " . . . . . . . | " |
| LXV. | " . . . . . . . | " |
| LXVI. | " . . . . . . . | " |
| LXXI. | " . . . . . . . | Kali chromicum. |
| LXXXIX. | " . . . . . . . | Phosphorus. |
| XC. | " . . . . . . . | " |
| CXVII. | " . . . . . . . | Spongia. |
| CXVIII. | " . . . . . . . | " |

## *I.*—CRANIAL CAVITY.

| | | |
|---|---|---|
| LXIX. | Hydrocephalus acutus, . . | Ferrum jod. |

## *K.*—PECTORAL CAVITY.

| | | |
|---|---|---|
| XLIX. | Broncho-Pneumonia, . . . | Carb. veg. |
| LXXVII. | Catarrh with hoarseness, . . | Kal. chrom. |
| XCI. | Bronchitis capillaris, . . . | Phosphor. |
| XCIII. | Phthisis incipiens, . . . | " |
| XCII. | Bronchitis, . . . . . | " |

## *L.*—ABDOMINAL CAVITY.

### GENERAL SCROFULOSIS.

| | | |
|---|---|---|
| XI. | Atrophia infant., . . . . | Arsen. |
| XII. | " " . . . . . | " |
| XVIII. | " " . . . . | Baryt. mur. |
| XIX. | Atrophia, . . . . . . | " " |
| XXIII. | " . . . . . . . . | Calc. carb. |
| XLVIII. | " . . . . . . . . | Carb. veg. |
| LI. | " . . . . . . . . | Dulcamara. |
| XCII. | Scarlatina scrof., . . . . | Phosphor. |
| XCIV. | General scrofulosis, . . . | " |
| CXVI. | Convulsions of scrof. children, . | Silicea. |
| CXIX. | General scrofulosis, . . . | Sulphur. |
| CXXVI. | Atrophia, . . . . . . | " |
| CXXVII. | General scrofulosis, . . . | " |

www.ingramcontent.com/pod-product-compliance
Lightning Source LLC
LaVergne TN
LVHW020056110826
845151LV00005B/1491

* 9 7 8 1 4 2 5 5 2 1 8 9 9 *